Preface

I am exceedingly pleased that Greyden Press is reprinting this historic and major classic work, Nursing and Anthropology: Two Worlds to Blend. This book was written in the mid-1960's and published in 1970. It was the first book to carve a pathway to the development of the field of transcultural nursing as a formal area of study and practice. The content in this book provides some of the epistemic knowledge and ontologic foundations for transcultural nursing from nursing and anthropology.

Developing a new body of transcultural nursing knowledge was a major challenge in nursing as it was a different way of knowing and understanding people. There were, however, several common interest and research areas to link or blend aspects of nursing and anthropology. This complementary linkage has remained active among its participants over the past 35 years and has greatly enriched both disciplines. This book has remained in great demand because it was the foundational book to establish the field of transcultural nursing.

Since 1970, the first definitive and substantial book, entitled Transcultural Nursing, Concepts, Theory, and Practice was published by J. Wiley in 1978 and the second edition in 1994 by Greyden Press (1994). These publications reflect how much transcultural nursing has become known and valued worldwide. Nursing and Anthropology has especially helped nursing students to understand the "roots", rationale for, and general development of transcultural nursing as an essential area of study and practice. It has also helped nurses and anthropologists to realize that transcultural nursing is not the same as anthropology, but rather two distinct disciplines whose scholars appreciate the commonalities and differences as well as the ways each discipline can make significant contributions.

In general, nursing students have found <u>Nursing and Anthropology</u> a most valuable historical book in the development of transcultural nursing. It is an early landmark book that helped move beyond the traditional medical model to some entirely new and different ideas in nursing. Such changes have been rewarding to see over the past four decades. For these reasons and others, this book remains a significant piece of work and as an exemplary model of how to establish a new field of study within a discipline and profession. With many requests of nurses and others, I feel confident that these nurses and others will welcome the availability of the book. I am most grateful to Rebecca Ensign of Greyden Press for her insight and eagerness to reprint this book.

Madeleine Leininger, Ph.D., L.H.D., D.S., C.T.N., R.N., F.A.A.N.
Author, 1994

Nursing and Anthropology: Two Worlds to Blend

Madeleine M. Leininger, R. N., Ph.D.

Greyden Press
Columbus, Ohio

Introduction

The world of man has always been an intriguing study for anthropologists and for students interested in discovering the essential nature of man's behaviour and ways of living. Today this study of man is more crucial than ever before, for it is needed in order to understand how men with different skin colors and different cultural backgrounds can live and work together in relative harmony. Currently, there are many stereotype responses, longstanding attitude sets, and behavior expectations shaping our relations with people whose skins may be brown, black, yellow, or red. As one looks beyond the color of the skin and interacts with these individuals or groups, one soon discovers the substantive core and the significant features of man's humanness and his behavioral dispositions. A sensitivity to and a knowledge of the similarities and differences between people with different cultural backgrounds is extremely important in establishing effective relationships and communications with others.

Culture is the blueprint for man's way of living, and only by understanding culture can we hope to gain the fullest understanding of man as a social and cultural being. It is the author's contention that in our efforts to understand intra-cultural and cross-cultural patterns we can no longer deny that cultural differences and similarities exist among men. Such understanding is one of the most crucial challenges of this decade. Cultural differences are often the basis for poor communication, interpersonal tensions, and hesitation in working effectively with others. Cultural similarities make us appreciate humanness, common human bonds, and behavior features which point to human universality. Both cultural differences and similarities challenge the student of human behavior to consider why men differ or are similar—one of the major riddles of life.

There has probably never been more open challenging of ideas, attitudes, beliefs, and behavior in relation to other ways of life than there is today. These challenges and confrontations have taken place on personal, social, political, psychological, economical, and cultural levels and largely in the pursuit of individual, group, or national interests. Unfortunately, these confrontations have not always been tempered with a knowledge of man's cultural history, his values, his beliefs, and his general patterns of living; and the consequence has been a frustrating impasse in communication and irritation with unfamiliar modes of thinking, acting, and reacting. In addition, many people show only limited interest and sometimes even unwillingness to attentively listen to and carefully observe another individual or his cultural group. Both the knowledge for understanding other people and a genuine interest in others are necessary for reciprocal learning and positive interpersonal experiences to take place in a cross-cultural situation. Maintaining an open attitude in examining one's own prejudices, attitudes and stereotyped perceptions is essential to learning about other people from other cultures.

Understanding people from different cultures can be one of the most exciting of all human experiences. This understanding and the understanding of subcultures in our own country is imperative for our development and survival, and for achievement of many social, political, educational, economical, and health goals. Gaps in knowledge about other people as well as a limited desire to understand people with different cultural backgrounds have throughout the history of man caused international tensions, wars, and a host of interpersonal stresses. The crucial problem is whether people will accept both the challenge and the responsibility of learning about the other peoples in the world with sufficient depth of knowledge and openness of mind to ease world tensions to discover new ways of living together. Certainly, this need is apparent if ever we wish for a modicum of world peace.

In the course of interacting with others, we discover that people live essentially in two worlds. There is the small personal world of the individual man, which is concerned with his day-to-day interactions with people in his immediate work and home environments. And then, there is the large impersonal world, which man knows about mainly through mass communication media and encounters with people in the course of his travel and business experiences. Man unconsciously struggles to "make sense" out of these two worlds, and to put them into a meaningful relationship. As he seeks to understand them, he is concerned with the question of why men differ in their beliefs, values, and behavior modes. This perplexing question continues to keep anthropologists and other interested social scientists intensely involved in a variety of research studies. Man tends to seek for a congruence of knowledge about people in his small and large worlds. The incongruencies, too, keep the scientist and non-scientist in search for answers or explanations.

There is a dearth of material dealing with cultural similarities and differences in nursing care practices. Consequently, there is much to learn not only about cultural similarities and differences, but also about how cultural factors influence the health and illness states of people in a society. Granted that some nurses have been exposed to the idea that cultural factors play a role in health maintenance and illness, many nurses have only a meager understanding of man's culture behavior and its relationship to health and illness. Knowledge of the health-illness system of different cultures is virtually a new area of study. In the past, nursing has given primary emphasis to the physical and psychological needs of people; the social and cultural aspects related to health and illness were perceived as less important. In fact, some nurses contended that the cultural and social aspects of health and illness belonged to social scientists.

Fortunately, a core of nurses is convinced that cultural and social factors are an integral part of nursing care and cannot be ruthlessly dissected from the physical and psychological dimensions of patient care and treatment. It will be interesting to see if in the future only lip service will be given to the cultural and social health needs of people, or if there will be a concerted effort to treat these factors as an essential part of patient care. Presently, as one reviews many nursing care plans, one is struck by the absence of any consideration of the patient's social and cultural needs. And frequently, when these factors are brought into the conference discussions, they are viewed as "last minute" considerations, "special additives," or "unexpected discoveries."

Currently, there is an interesting dictum found in nursing which states that "nursing is concerned with man's bio-psycho-social needs." This shorthand expression reflects the current areas of emphasis in nursing, and reflects the omission of cultural aspects from nursing practice. Some nurses contend that the term "social" includes "cultural," as if man's cultural needs were subsumed under the social and were synonymous with it. But as one pursues the subject further with these professional nurses, one discovers that they have only a limited understanding of the concept of culture and that they show limited evidence of incorporating cultural aspects into patient care or the teaching of students. There is an urgent need to make cultural and other anthropological concepts a part of the nurse's thinking so that clients can have their cultural needs understood and met.

During the past five years, the author has been working closely with professional nurses and students in service and educational settings. On undergraduate and graduate levels she has introduced perspectives on the interrelationships of anthropology and nursing. A yearly seminar entitled "Anthropology and Nursing" was designed to explore several theories, problems, issues, and research possibilities in the fields of nursing and anthropology. Positive and highly rewarding experiences from the teaching of these courses have provided much valuable knowledge for the contents in this book. In addition, the author's consultation and group discussion experiences in a variety of health and university settings across the country provided other insights about the usefulness of anthropological concepts in the health fields. The author is grateful to her students, teachers and professional staff who have eagerly, candidly, and imaginatively offered their views on the subject. As a consequence, the book reflects the active thinking and interest of many students and colleagues who were eager to explore the relationships between health and social science fields.

The purpose of the book is to facilitate a rapprochement between the fields of nursing and anthropology, so that each discipline will benefit from the contribution of the other. But, most importantly, the book has been designed to stimulate nurses so that they will blend together nursing knowledge and relevant anthropological concepts to ensure that people will receive good nursing care. It is anticipated that, in future years, as nurses and anthropologists work together they will refine, deepen, and expand the ideas presented in this book, and hopefully generate many new operational concepts. The author hopes that this book will stimulate further developments in research, teaching, and practice among nurses and anthropologists.

The theme of the book, "Two Worlds to Blend," is that the fields of anthropology and nursing must be interdigitated so that each field will profit from the contribution of the other. Currently, there is the one world of nursing which is striving to understand man's behavior and health needs so that there will be improvements in nursing practice. And there is the other world of anthropology, which continues to gain many new insights into man's behavior through the course of time and in different places. It is apparent that if these two fields were sharing their special knowledge and experiences, both would undoubtedly see new pathways in thinking and research. To many nurses, anthropology is a vague field and is irrelevant to nursing; to many anthropologists, nurses are hard-working and busy persons who seldom have time for intellectual and research inquiry. In order to change these perceptions, there is a need to bring the people in these two worlds closer together so that there will be a fruitful fusion, one which will generate some new ideas for future scientific and humanistic endeavors.

The field of nursing is growing rapidly and is extending its traditional boundaries of health practice and education. Nurses today are working with people in a variety of communities and world settings and they need to have an understanding of the particular needs of people of different cultures and subcultural backgrounds. The new thrust of community-centered nursing which focused upon understanding man's community health needs is gaining momentum. Nurses are generally eager to learn new ideas, to interact with different people, and to face new challenges to improve patient care, and so they will undoubtedly recognize more and more the relevance of anthropological concepts to community health nursing practices. As new leaders emerge into the nursing field with broad academic backgrounds in the natural and social sciences, they will also be ready to establish creative practices so that the cultural and social health needs of clients will be met.

Contents

1 The Two Worlds and the Nature of Anthropology — 1
   The Two Worlds — 1
   Anthropology: Nature, Goals and Interests — 4
   The Subfields of Anthropology — 9
   Anthropology: Basic and Applied — 14

2 The Potential Contribution of Anthropology to Nursing — 17

3 The Nature of Nursing and Its Contribution to Anthropology — 28
   The Nature of Nursing: The Author's Conception — 28
   Contributions of Nursing to Anthropology — 33
   Facts and Hunches about the Delayed Interest of Nursing in Anthropology — 37

4 The Culture Concept and American Culture Values in Nursing — 45
   A New Dimension for Nursing — 47
   The Meaning of the Culture Concept — 48
   Manifest and Ideal Culture — 50
   Culture and Subculture — 50
   American Cultural Values and Nursing — 51

5 The Traditional Culture of Nursing and the Emerging New One — 63

Other-Directed and Self-Directed Behaviors — 65
Paternalism, Self-Sacrifice, and Self-Needs — 67
Authoritarian and Democratic Values — 70
Doing Versus Intellectual Norms — 72
Uniformity and Diversity — 74
Practicality and High Idealism — 75
Focus of Care — 76
Role Behavior — 77
Symbolic Crutches — 78
Personality Attributes and "Professionalism" — 79

6 Cultural Differences Between Patient and Staff and Their Influence on Patient Care — 83

Understanding Cultural Differences: The Key to Success — 83
Reasons for the Neglect of Key Questions — 84
Patient-Staff Study Situations — 86
   Study One: German-American Patient — 86
   Study Two: Italian-American Child — 90
   Study Three: Spanish-Speaking Patient Group — 91
   Study Four: Afro-American Patient — 94

7 The Use of Cultural Factors in Patient Care: Examples from Different Cultures — 97

Ways to Gain Cultural Awareness — 97
Understanding Culture Factors as a Basis for Patient Care — 99
Cultural Factors in Patient-Care Situations — 101
   Situation One: Czech-American Patient — 101
   Situation Two: Mexican-American Patient — 103
   Situation Three: Afro-American Patient — 104
   Situation Four: Swedish-American Patient — 106
   Situation Five: Cheyenne Indian and Anglo-American Couple — 107

8 The Cultural Context of Behavior: Spanish-Americans and Nursing Care — 111

Meaning of the Cultural Context of Behavior — 111
The Cultural Context of the Spanish-American — 112
   General Cultural Features — 112
   Social and Kinship Aspects — 113
   Religious Aspects — 114
   Political Aspects — 115
   Economic Aspects — 115
   Health-Illness Systems — 117
Implications for Nursing — 121

9 An Adopted Vietnamese Child: A Cultural Shock — 128

Guest Co-Author: Charlotte Heidema, R.N., M.S.

Stevie: the Adopted Child — 128
Stevie's New World — 129
The Adopted Parents and Their Anticipation of a Son — 130
The Family Adjustment — 131
Nurse-Family Relationship as Experienced
  by the Nurse Therapist — 133
A Comparison of the Two Cultures — 134
   Culture History Aspects and the Cultural Context — 135
   Sociocultural, Economic, and Kinship Factors — 135
   Vietnamese Socialization Processes — 136
   American Culture and Socialization Values — 137
Inferences from the Cultural Data Regarding Stevie — 138
Nursing Plan for Future Situation like Stevie's Case — 140

10 Health Institutions as Cultural and Social Systems — 145

Basic Definitions of Social and Cultural Systems — 146
   Formal and Informal Systems — 147
   Open and Closed Systems — 148
   Macro and Micro Systems — 149
Three Dimensions for Studying Sociocultural Systems — 149

Components of a Sociocultural System 152
Conceptions and Misconceptions
 about Sociocultural Systems 154
Static and Dynamic Systems 154
Eufunctional and Dysfunctional Systems 154
Patient-Staff Socialization 156
Hospitals as a Replica of the Community 157
Role-taking: Static and Dynamic Aspects 158
Nurses' Perceptions of Sociocultural
 Systems 159
The Culture of the Hospital 161

11 Ethnoscience: A Promising Research Approach to Improve Nursing Practice 167

The Patient's View of Illness Is Important 168
Ethnoscience: Definition and Goals 168
Assumptions, Principles, and Theoretical Views of
 Ethnoscience 170
Application of the Method: Gadsup Health Practitioner
 Roles 172
Merits of the Ethnoscience Method 175

Index 179

Nursing and Anthropology:
Two Worlds to Blend

1.1 The Two Worlds and the Nature of Anthropology

The Two Worlds

Nursing and anthropology are two fascinating and important fields whose students are interested in the behavior of man and in man's current and future well being.* These fields appear to be two different worlds, and yet they have bonds of mutual interest that support and reinforce each other. Both nursing and anthropology support the holistic concept of man and have quite similar philosophical and theoretical interests. Although both disciplines have their own special problems for investigation, there are methods of studying human behavior which could be extremely fruitful to nurses and anthropologists alike. It is rather strange that nursing and anthropology have been largely orbiting in their own spheres for many years, with only limited awareness of and interest in each others' fields and contributions to mankind. The perplexing question is why the people in these two fields have not shared their special insights, theoretical interests, and practical skills with one another through the years. Interestingly enough, each discipline began at approximately the same time (the mid-nineteenth century); and yet, there has been no serious interdisciplinary interest until quite recently.

---

*The word "man" will be used in this book to refer to man as a generalized being, including women and children.

2 The Two Worlds and the Nature of Anthropology

In the examination of these two worlds, one finds a number of similarities as well as a number of differences. The world of anthropology is much more comprehensive in its scope and interests than the field of nursing. The field of nursing is concerned essentially with the health and illness problems and behavior of man over a relatively short span of time. In contrast, anthropology maintains an extremely broad interest in man's health and illness behavior over thousands of years, and sees these aspects from an evolutionary and functional perspective. Both fields, however, share common interests in their desire to understand the multiple forces that threaten or support man's health status.

Nursing and anthropology each have their own "field focus." Nursing has traditionally used an institutional clinical focus patterned upon the medical model; recently, however, the focus is becoming extended and approximates the anthropologist's broad field or community-study approach. With the emerging interest of nursing in the community field-study method, there is promise of reciprocal research and practice field areas. Undoubtedly ethnographic methods of studying whole or partial communities will be found useful in nursing. The field-study method encourages professional workers to study people by fairly continuous interaction with, and systematic observation of people in their familiar and natural settings. Naturalistic participant-observation is the traditional method of anthropology, and is beginning to be used by nurse researchers. This method provides opportunities to study the recurrent and non-recurrent life experiences of people and the factors related to human viability and longevity. Both nursing and anthropology are vitally interested in the importance of primary data and in collecting their own data directly from the people and in the people's own verbatim statements and explanations. The desire for "live" data of a descriptive nature is believed to be extremely important for obtaining an accurate picture of the human way of life.

Both nursing and anthropology are interested in a single, specific, and unitary whole. For the nurse this is the individual person or the family unit; for the anthropologist it is a specific unit of any size. As the nurse and the anthropologist study or work with a specific whole, they both rely heavily upon direct observations and communications with people in each unit. They both may employ similar approaches in explaining the phenomena under study by the use of similar explanatory models about human behavior. The use of functional models to explain human behavior supports the view that behavior should be interpreted with reference to the entire unit as an integrated and whole entity, and not from only certain aspects of that total entity. Though only a few nurses have had preparation in using the various functional explanatory models found in anthropology, one can predict they will use them more in the future and find them helpful in explaining behavior.

Recently, there have been signs of heightened interest in blending the two worlds of nursing and anthropology. Much of this interest has emanated from a small group of nurse-anthropologists and anthropologists who are maintaining an active interest in both fields. They are convinced that each discipline has much to offer the other, but that there is an initial need to explore areas of common interest and to tap new areas that have potential benefits for one another. Lately there have been some nursing students who are taking anthropology courses and are finding that anthropological concepts, theories, and research methods have relevance for nursing. These students have been particularly excited about how the broad and multi-faceted framework anthropology leads to an understanding of healthy and sick persons. It is the culture concept and an understanding of the cultural background of people that courts these students' interest and makes them realize what knowledge areas have been missing in the past to fully understand patients' needs. There are also a few anthropologists employed in schools of nursing and in health centers who are asking penetrating and relevant questions in order to help nurses understand the cultural significance and validity of their teaching content, research approaches, and patient practices. These anthropologists provide a fresh perspective about nursing which leads nurses to new dimensions of thought. At the same time, the anthropologists are learning much about nurses and the nursing profession, and are sharing these observations with nurses and colleagues.

Anthropological knowledge is essential to nurses in their sincere efforts to improve patient (or client) care by understanding the cultural stresses and factors affecting his health state. Anthropology as a humanistic and scientific field has remained vitally interested in the health and illness behavior of different cultural groups, and it is this knowledge which should form the basis for understanding and planning peoples' health needs and problems. The variations between different cultural groups in maintaining a state of well being or in perpetuating a state of illness are known to anthropologists, and this information makes the nurse realize that health and illness are largely culturally derived.

In some cultures it is the expected norm to exhibit certain kinds of illness-like behavior, and members of the health professions must not be too hasty to eradicate or suppress this illness unless they understand cultural factors affecting this behavioral expression. In another culture, illness may be frought with considerable anxiety and all efforts taken to immediately and effectively eradicate the ailment. Thus one can begin to see that the ambitious and good intentional desires of nurses and physicians to quickly and effectively eradicate all signs of disease or illness, may be a highly questionable practice for some cultural groups. These groups are quite capable of challenging our good and noble efforts. Moreover, it probably never occurred to nurses that in some cultures hyperactivity and masochism are part of the "normal" established way of life and that this behavior helps to perpetuate the culture. These examples and others make us realize that *health and illness are an integral part of man's cultural way of life.* Health and illness are closely interwoven aspects of man's cultural values, beliefs and practices. This broad cultural frame of reference extends the nurse's understanding of the multiple factors involved in man's behavior, and puts her in a favorable position to make decisions about what people need to help them live in their culture.

Accordingly, anthropologists can benefit from the experiences of nurses with sick and well people, and especially, from their experiences with people under the extreme stress conditions related to death, unexpected life experiences, or the traumas of new treatments and unfamiliar care practices. As the nurse works with people facing the threat of death, severe pain, or a variety of other stresses, she observes their capacity for adapting. Although anthropologists have long been interested in man's ability to endure stress and in the mechanisms he uses to survive, he can benefit from the nurse's observations and interpretations of the clients' behavior. In fact, the anthropologist may obtain special knowledge and new insight about stress and human behavior from the nurse. The anthropologist could well ask certain questions of the nurse and explore them with her: 1) Under undue stress, what is revealed about man's general adaptation abilities? 2) What can be predicted about man's evolutionary and physical development in light of his sickness-wellness adaptation potential? 3) In light of different kinds of illnesses and the nurse's nurturant practices, what can be said about man's rehabilitation potential? 4) What kinds of illnesses show less or more responsiveness to the nurturant activities of the nurse?

Anthropology: Nature, Goals, and Interests

Anthropology is the science of man, which seeks to discover man's ways of living, ways of believing, and ways of adapting to changing circumstances in his human (physical, psychological, cultural, and social) environments. It is a descriptive and comparative science which attempts to discover the answer to the question, what is man? The word "anthropology" is derived from the Greek words, *anthropos*, "man," and *logos*, "study;" it thus translated means "man-study." The central focus of anthropology is on understanding man and mankind. Anthropologists are deeply interested in studying man in our modern society, and man as he has lived in the past in diverse places around the world. Most important, anthropologists are interested in the way man has adapted to and maintained himself in different physical and cultural environments.

It is only natural that human beings are curious about man's origin, his past modes of living, and his ways of surviving through time. Man is, indeed, a very old and unique being who has learned to make his own tools, to obtain food, and to survive in some rather precarious environments. Man has also proved capable of creating his own cultural norms and his own social and political forms of organization in order for groups of people to live together. Man is a marvelous being, and much of our knowledge about him as a physical, cultural, and social being has come from anthropological writings and investigations. However, there is still much to learn about man. Anthropologists continue to work for a scientific, humanistic and comprehensive knowledge about man, so that they can explain, interpret, and predict cross-cultural human behavior.

Anthropology is both a scientific and a humanistic field which is concerned with man's long-range development from the time when there were many different species of pre-man to the present when there is one species, *homo sapiens*. Since man has been evolving as a species for approximately one million years, there is a variety of interesting and informative findings which make us appreciate his special development. Physically, socially, and culturally, man has changed greatly through time, and he will undoubtedly continue to change in future years.

Although other disciplines are interested in and contribute to the scientific study of man, *anthropology is the only discipline which takes a comprehensive and longitudinal look at man.* This means that man is viewed from multi-faceted dimensions and from a time and space perspective. For anthropologists, scientific interest in man relates not only to the present and the past, but also to the continuing forces which have shaped and will continue to shape man's cultural development. The anthropological insights gained from the study of man in the most remote places in the world, in the streets of our present-day cities, and in modern rural areas, provide a unique comparative view of man. They disclose man's capacity to live in varying kinds of environments and under the influence of diverse forces. No other field of scientific endeavor seems to offer such breadth of knowledge and such rich and intimate data about man, as does the field of anthropology.

The anthropological approach to the study of man requires that the anthropologist live with the people he is studying. The opportunity to live among people with a different way of life provides both invaluable knowledge about the group of people under study and a fresh perspective on the anthropologist's own way of living. The anthropologist needs to exhibit a considerable degree of patience, empathy, and compassion if the people's indigenous ideas and practices are to come to the foreground. In return, a skilled anthropologist usually obtains much descriptive and detailed data about the people and they share this knowledge with many disciplines which are concerned with man's behavior and ways of living.

Anthropologists generally do not remove people from their natural and familiar living environments to some artificial laboratory setting in order to study them. The principal anthropological method of studying people, called the *field-study community method*, requires that anthropologists live with the people in their natural cultural and physical environment, and provides special opportunities not common to other scientists. This naturalistic study approach helps the anthropologist to understand how people actually live in their familiar day-to-day setting, and what constitutes their daily, monthly, and yearly activities. As a consequence, many rich, detailed and special facts about the people are discovered, which are rarely obtained in a laboratory situation or when one "drops in or out" of a village or community. Spontaneous actions, slips of the tongue, casual behavior, conflicts, and crisis situations can be observed as one lives with people over an extended period of time. In sum, anthropological data about a designated group's life style tends to be more valid and reliable than the data obtained by scientists who remove people from their natural life settings or markedly modify their usual way of life in order to study them.

Man's culture is both material and non-material. "Material culture" refers to all the man-made objects found in association with a given cultural group, whereas "nonmaterial culture" refers to those other aspects of the culture which are not material in nature and form. Accordingly, man possesses many symbolic referents which the anthropologist must study to appreciate the concepts of man and his culture. Man's symbolic referents and values, and the other material and non-material aspects of culture, have special meaning and significance as one studies man in his broad cultural and ecological context. Most importantly, anthropologists must seek to understand man's total cultural forms and their special meanings in order to comprehend man as he exists in his own cultural setting. It is knowledge of the *wholeness* of man's behavior which anthropologists strive to obtain. DeLaguna states that, "Anthropology is the only discipline that offers a conceptual schema for the whole context of human experiences."[1] This statement implies that anthropology endeavors to discover and understand many different parts of a whole culture and how these cultural parts are interrelated with each other, so that a total picture of the people develops. Not all parts of the culture are equally significant, nor does one need to know every part of the culture before one can understand it. However, one tries to get a broad view of as many aspects of the culture as is possible in order to see how and why the culture functions and exists as it does. Thus a careful study of the material and non-material culture and of the interrelationship of the different parts of a culture is important as a means to determine how the people have lived, worked, and survived within their own culture. Understanding the many parts of man's culture helps to know the totality of man's world.

Most anthropologists hold that anthropology is a social science but there are those who disagree. DeLaguna, for example, contends that anthropology is not a social science:

> The true social sciences are intense explorations into compartmentalized areas of human activity, where understanding of certain things is achieved by ignoring the rest. Yet, if we have learned anything, it is that all parts of a culture must be understood together, that the context and interrelationships are more essential than the specific parts, no matter how well the latter are known. Let us not trade the heritage of this insight, no matter how unlikely of complete attainment, for the certainty of half a loaf.[2]

DeLaguna's position is to emphasize the importance of understanding the relationships between all parts of a culture rather than limiting one's study to a very limited and specialized aspect.

Through the years, anthropology has become recognized as a *unifying science* which synthesizes man's behavior and evolution. Unlike some disciplines which deal repeatedly with restricted and isolated segments of man's behavior and life activities, anthropology is a discipline which emphasizes that man's behavior must be seen as extending through a continuous life stream and in the frame of his cultural context. Moreover, his behavior, beliefs, and values, must be viewed from the totality of his life experiences. From this comprehensive and unified view special aspects of man can also be studied in depth in the subfields of anthropology such as linguistic anthropology, physical anthropology and psychological anthropology. Both generalized anthropology and specialized areas of anthropology are features of the field. Herskovits, a cultural anthropologist, contends that anthropology has a far wider breadth of interest in its pursuit of understanding man than do related fields in the social sciences and the humanities.[3]

As a scientific discipline, anthropology is interested in man's history and in the multiple forces from his cultural past which have led him to his present ways. The Australian Aborigine, who lives in a non-technological society and a harsh natural environment, is as important an area of study in furthering a broad understanding of man as is contemporary Western man, who lives in a highly technological modern world. This comparative view of societies helps us to appreciate man's achievements and his adaptative abilities. It gives us ways to predict man's future directions and the multiple dynamic forces that continue influencing his destiny and future opportunities. In general, we may view man as a highly successful being who in the course of time has withstood many rugged stress and adaptation situations. Man has lived for almost one million years—a testimony to his tenacity. He has had to cope with many unusual trials to ensure his physical survival, and he has also dealt with strange political, social, and economic problems. Most important, he has devised cultural norms which have served as important guidelines for his social development and survival. Man's trial for success in living and survival, however, is far from complete. Today he is facing some entirely new challenges and different kinds of living and adaptation stresses. If he is to survive, he must once again cope with new forces and must develop ways to avoid annihilating himself and the life resources which he is dependent upon for survival.

For a long time, anthropologists have been interested in the network of social relations that man develops and maintains within a particular culture. Man has learned not only to adjust to different sets of social relations, but also to participate in social groups to further the full development both of himself and of the groups in their own right. Social groups are the important viable units into which each man is born, and they stimulate individuals to become active group participants for the sake of their own social, cultural, and biological well-being. Social institutions, each of which integrates a network of organized social relations between persons whose activities and interests are thereby organized to meet specific human problems and needs, are also important to man. In fact, practically everything man does occurs in relation to social institutions. Within these institutions, one finds groups of people governed by implicit or explicit cultural rules or by established expectations of one another. There are also symbolic referents for the purpose of guiding one's behavior, activities, and goals. Man spends his entire life in social groups and institutions which are important to man's full human development.

The ultimate scientific and humanistic goal of anthropology is to accurately describe, explain, and predict man's behavior from a cross-cultural perspective. Anthropologists are searching for universal and particularistic features of human behavior in diverse places and throughout the long history of man. And from comparative studies, generalizations can be made and then tested to explain and predict man's behavior. To date, anthropologists have systematically studied a number of different cultures from a comparative viewpoint. They have identified several factors which tend to influence the variability in man's behavior and existence, such as his constitutional endowment, his special cultural rules of behavior, his psychological disposition, and the type of social organization he supports. Anthropologists have also identified the ways in which man responds to outside cultural groups and to forced or gradual contacts with other cultures. They have identified different kinds of processes related to culture change.

Currently, there are many interesting theories and speculations about man's behavior, but many of these theories still need to be subjected to rigorous scrutiny in relation to a variety of cultures. Since anthropology is less than one hundred years old, it is a relatively new field accumulating many observations and theories which must be verified or rejected in the future. At present, many old theories are being re-examined and many new theories are being subjected to preliminary scientific examination. Man has been studied all over the world, but there are still a few places where he has not been studied. The interest in finding cultural groups which have not been studied remains high, as does interest in restudying known cultures. Today, it is difficult for anthropologists to offer a universal theory about man's behavior because of the wide variations about human behavior which are contingent upon environmental and human situations. However, the ideal goal of anthropology is to state both universal and particularistic laws governing man's behavior.

In the on-going pursuit of the study of man, new mathematical methods, cybernetic models, cross-cultural testing techniques, computer methods, and the ethnoscience approach are valuable methods to increase the reliability and validity of anthropological findings. These tools should help the anthropologist accelerate his work of testing theories and making predictive generalizations about man.

The Subfields of Anthropology

In a scientific and humanistic discipline where there is an explosion of knowledge and concomitant specialization of interests, one will find subfields developing within the general field. This is only to be expected, since scientific problems require depth analysis and detailed scrutiny. Since specialization is the process of focusing-in on an area of study, each scientist must take extra time to keep informed of the general knowledge in his field. Accordingly, anthropologists must keep abreast of the general findings, theories, and research goals in the field, but must also become specialists by studying a subfield of anthropology. Some subfields are closely related to one another, and so the research findings from these subfields bear upon one another significantly. Physical anthropology and archaeology, for example, are closely aligned to each other. The principal subfields of anthropology are physical anthropology, archaeology, cultural anthropology (and general ethnology), social anthropology, psychological anthropology, and linguistic anthropology. Each of these subfields has its own special body of knowledge, and its own research focus, methods, and goals. We shall briefly discuss these subfields below.

The subfield of *physical anthropology* focuses upon the origin and development of man as a physical and biological organism. Physical anthropologists are interested in what man has been in the past, how he became what he is, what he is today, and what he will become in the future. They study evolutionary changes and population differences. An earlier emphasis in physical anthropology was on the measurement of the human body and upon describing and classifying human physical types. In recent years, the focus has been on human genetics, in relation to which the physical anthropologists investigate the genetic base of man's physical manifestations, the expression and fate of genes in populations, and the genetic basis of human evolution. Human populations in relation to their ecological, social, and cultural setting are studied by physical anthropologists. In general, one can say that physical anthropologists focus upon the study of man's origin and development through the course of time by studying his physical, genetic, and morphological characteristics in relation to his ecological and cultural settings.

Physical anthropologists find it difficult to discriminate sharply between geographic populations and ethnic subdivisions, as there are a series of gradual variations within these human population groups. Labels are often used to distinguish major population groups and ethnic subdivisions; however these labels are often misinterpreted by lay people to ascribe racial and hereditary inferiorities or superiorities to different population groups. Physical expressions of populations are more precisely found as *genetic variations* between the total population groups rather than in a specific label such as "yellow people." Since physical anthropologists deal with the biological and genetic aspects of man, they may be found working at the universities in collaboration with the staffs in the departments of anatomy and physiology and with faculty and students in medicine, nursing, and dentistry. They also work closely with geneticists in studying human breeding, and with zoologists and paleontologists in studying the relation of man to other animals.

Currently one can find such specialization areas within the field of physical anthropology as human genetics, primatology, human paleontology (or paleoanthropology), growth and development, blood groups and types, constitutional relationships, and comparative human physiology. It is anticipated that health personnel in the future will be working more closely with physical anthropologists because of their mutual interest areas, particularly in regard to human development, physiology, and genetics.

Archaeology or prehistory, is a study of ancient peoples and their culture and technology. Archaeology approaches man's prehistory with the goal of discovering man's culture as it existed in times long before writing and written records. Archaeologists have studied man before written records were available as well as since writing and records have existed. They are interested in the past ways man lived and get such information by carefully excavating the remains and studying man-made material cultures, such as temples, dwellings, and old ruins. They analyze man's living sites, his tools, his fossil remains, and any other evidences of his culture and technology. As these scientists unearth objects by their special methods and techniques, they discover various phases and sequences relating to how man lived in the distant past and how he developed different technological tools. From this data, archaeologists can not only learn about the unwritten history of a past culture, but they also obtain data from which to make inferences about the people's social organization, religion, and cultural behavior. Prehistoric tools, objects, and other artifacts are interpreted in the light of different theories about man and his cultural life, and in relation to other evidence available about the particular excavation site and cultural area. Many new discoveries and important findings about early man become known to us through the careful and systematic work of archaeologists. Their work is tedious and difficult and it often requires many years of studying a particular archaeological site or cultural area.

Two kinds of archaeology are often referred to in the literature, namely, anthropological archaeology and classical archaeology. Anthropological archaeology has been described above as the work of the scientific prehistorian who studies past extinct cultures or past phases of our present-day culture. Classical archaeology is usually the work of a historian rather than an anthropologist, who studies written records or documents such as those of ancient Egypt or Greece.

Cultural anthropology refers to the description and analysis of the life practices and the rules of behavior of a particular cultural group. Cultural anthropologists are concerned generally with the non-biological aspects of man, or the general way of life of a designated group of people. In subsequent chapters, there will be a full discussion of the culture concept; for the present, we can speak broadly of *culture* as referring to the *total complex of material objects, tools, ideas, organizations, and all material and non-material aspects related to man's existence.* The cultural anthropologist is particularly interested in studying diverse human cultures in various places in the world, and in accounting for the similarities and differences between men in terms of their various cultural beliefs, values, and ways of living. These scientists also study the material aspects of a culture, such as technologies. They study all forms of non-material culture, such as religion, art, music, economics, political behavior, social organization, ceremonial life, kinship and marriage patterns, and symbolic forms of communication.

Ethnographies are usually considered an integral and important part of the work of both cultural and social anthropologists. An *ethnography* is a factual description of the way of life of a specific group of people. For example, a cultural anthropologist may derive an ethnography of the Sioux Indians or of the Samoans. American anthropologists tend to speak of themselves as "cultural anthropologists," in contrast to the British anthropologists who say that they are "social ethnographers" or "social anthropologists." Both types of anthropologists produce ethnographies of cultural groups, even though their method and focus may differ slightly. Some cultural anthropologists have special interest areas branching out from ethnology, and may function as ethnopsychologists, ethnosociologists, ethnophysiologists, ethnomusicologists, and/or general ethnographers.

During the early part of the twentieth century a new trend in anthropology developed, and the subfield of social anthropology emerged primarily in England and France. Social anthropology is concerned with the scientific study and analysis of social structures, social groups, social institutions, and the social behavior of different peoples from a comparative point of view. Social anthropologists are primarily interested in developing theories and scientific generalizations about the different patterns of social interaction which comprise various social systems, and in different societies and their forms of social organizations and social structure. Social anthropologists emphasize the study of *social structures*—a term which refers to the various social, economic, political, kinship, and religious aspects of the life-ways of people in a given society. These scientists study the complex features and interrelationships of these various components of social structure. From their studies they arrive at generalizations about man's social behavior. Social anthropology takes a generalized approach to a comparative analysis of human behavior by critically examining theoretical problems related to social structure features, particularly the social organization of a given societal group in relation to its characteristic personality tendencies and cultural values. The term "ethnology" was at first used interchangeably with "social anthropology;" but today the term *ethnology* refers exclusively to the comparative analysis of societal groups with respect to their cultural and social history, forms of social organization, and general sociocultural behavior.

Frequently, students of human behavior ask if social anthropology and sociology are not the same. Although scientists in both these fields study a number of common problems, their goals, scope, analytic focus, and theoretical framework for explaining behavior are in general not the same. Even their approaches and methods of studying social problems differ in several respects.

Social anthropology deals with human social behavior in a wide cross-cultural perspective and over an extended period of time. Social anthropologists are interested in making scientific generalizations about social groups based upon different comparative aspects of social structure phenomena, such as the political, economic, kinship, religion, and social systems of two or more societies. They are interested in both Western and non-Western social structure features. In addition, social and psychological anthropologists are deeply interested in viewing socialization practices and child-rearing problems from a cross-cultural viewpoint. In contrast, sociologists take a much more limited focus and deal mostly with intrasocial problems, primarily in Western societies. They generally investigate a limited and highly specific social problem, and are not particularly concerned with the multifactors in a society which influence human behavior. Furthermore, their focus is not primarily upon the comparative social systems of Western and non-Western societies. Nonetheless, some collaboation exists between these disciplines. Lately, as each field becomes more specialized and auto-definitive in its goals, one finds that departments of social anthropology and sociology are becoming separated administratively, but still maintaining collaborative interest.

In the past, anthropologists have contended that *psychological anthropology* was an integral part of the subfield of social anthropology and not a distinct subfield in its own right. However, it is the belief of this author, along with a number of other anthropologists, that psychological anthropology is becoming a legitimate and special subfield in its own right. The content, problems, goals, and interests of psychological anthropology are becoming more specialized as these anthropologists delve into weighty problems related to such areas as personality development, socialization processes, individual and group behavior, mental illness and culture, psychocultural expressions of behavior, comparative behavior (viewed intra- and cross-culturally), and comparative child-rearing practices. New insights into these areas and many others are rapidly unfolding as psychological anthropologists work with other psychological anthropologists and with an array of miscellaneous specialists from different fields. Marked emphasis is given to theoretical underpinnings and cross-cultural generalizations which purport to explain human behavior from a personality, cultural, and societal viewpoint. The interrelationships between these three variables are critically analyzed by psychological anthropologists.

In general, psychological anthropologists are interested in the comparative analysis of cross-cultural socialization processes, personality manifestations (including the role, structure, and function of personality in a culture), psycholinguistic phenomena, the role of cultural values in personality formation, specific child-rearing variables and their relationship to social structure, evolutionary aspects of personality in relation to sociocultural dimensions, and mental health and culture. A number of psychological anthropologists are currently interested in studying and explaining the growing number of deviant personalities in our own culture, viewed in comparison to other Western and non-Western societies. This is a fascinating field, for it provides a broad integrative framework in which to understand man's total personality and behavior, which are viewed in far more limited terms by other personality and behavioral scientists.

Linguistic anthropology refers to the description and scientific analysis of the language of a given cultural group. Linguistic anthropologists are responsible for recording, studying, and carefully analyzing the vocabulary, sounds, and grammatical structures of the different languages of the world. After studying a particular language, they compare it with other languages to determine the structural and historical relationships among languages as well as the role of linguistic changes. Social, cultural, psychological, and physiological factors are studied in relation to the way they influence language expression. Language is necessary for transmitting culture from one generation to another and from one group or individual to another. In studying a culture, the linguistic anthropologist generally studies a culture which has no system of writing. Furthermore, there is no way of knowing the language except by living with a cultural group and studying their language. The linguistic anthropologist often collaborates with structural linguists in the development of valid ways to study and analyze the language of a particular cultural group.

The term "ethnolinguistics" is frequently mentioned by linguistic anthropologists; it refers to the systematic study of how language and culture are related to one another, as well as to the general approach to a study of the language of a particular indigenous group. There are two subdivisions of linguistics, namely *descriptive linguistics* and *comparative historical linguistics.* Descriptive linguistics focuses on the grammar, vocabulary, and sound system of a language, and how they function together to make a language entity. Comparative linguistics deals with the history, origin, and development of languages from a comparative viewpoint. A comparative linguist will generally trace the development of groups of related languages from a stem (or parent) language. Linguistic anthropology is rapidly becoming a highly scientific, respected, and important field. Its scientists are developing some unique methods to study rigorously the language systems of diverse cultures.

Anthropology: Basic and Applied

Anthropology, like other scientific fields, has scientists who are primarily interested in developing and examining theories which can be tested in the field. Their efforts are directed toward the discovery of new scientific knowledge about man or the verification of formerly highly speculative theories, without the primary goal of applying this knowledge to practical life problems. These scientists are often referred to as *basic or "pure" scientists*. Correspondingly, there are also scientists in the field who are *primarily* interested in applying anthropological knowledge to the solution of practical life problems, and these anthropologists are referred to as *applied anthropologists*. However, many of the so-called "applied" scientists are actively involved and interested in the activities of the "pure" scientists, so that a clear and distinct dichotomy is often difficult to support.

Since World War II, the demand for applied anthropologists in government, business, professional fields, international agencies, federal agencies, educational institutions, and military and civilian research departments has increased considerably. Our society continues to demand people who are willing to apply research knowledge to practical domestic, national, and international problems. In the course of functioning as an applied anthropologist, the scientist generally has opportunities to perform basic research studies or to combine pure and applied research interests. There is, consequently, a good bit of ambiguity as to whether any anthropologist is strictly "pure" or "applied." This author believes that the traditionally assumed dichotomous areas subdividing anthropology into pure and applied fields is becoming less definitive today.

FOOTNOTES

[1] Frederica DeLaguna, "Presidential Address—1967," *American Anthropologist*, Vol. 70, No. 3, June 1968, p. 475.
[2] *Ibid.*
[3] Melville J. Herskovits, *Cultural Anthropology*, New York: Alfred A. Knopf, 1955.

SUGGESTED REFERENCES

Beals, R. L., and Harry Hoijer, *Introduction to Anthropology*, Third Edition, New York: Macmillan Company, 1965.
Bohannon, Paul, *Social Anthropology*, New York: Holt, Rinehart, and Winston, 1963.
Cohen, Yehudi, Editor, *Man in Adaptation: The Cultural Present*, Chicago: Aldine Publishing Company, 1968.
Fried, Morton H., *Readings in Anthropology, Vol. I: Physical Anthropology, Linguistics, Archeology; Vol. II: Cultural Anthropology*, New York: Thomas Y. Crowell Company, 1959.
Hsu, Frances L. K., *Psychological Anthropology: Approach to Culture and Personality*, Illinois: The Dorsey Press, 1961.

Keesing, Felix M., *Cultural Anthropology: The Science of Custom*, New York: Holt, Rinehart, and Winston, 1965.
Mead, Margaret., *Anthropology: A Human Science*, New York: D. Van Nostrand Company, Inc., 1957.

2 The Potential Contribution of Anthropology To Nursing

If the Greek historian, Herodotus, known as the "father of anthropology," and Florence Nightingale, the "founder of modern professional nursing," had lived in the same era and had an on-going opportunity to discuss reciprocal relationships between the fields of anthropology and nursing, one might predict that their dialogue would have ended in a happy and successful marriage of the two fields. The two worlds of anthropology and nursing, however, continue to move in their own separate orbits. Nonetheless, practitioners in these two fields have similar interests in that they are concerned with the social and behavioral aspects of man's health status. Both Herodotus and Nightingale were interested in the kinds of stresses that man experienced and how he adapted to environmental forces. Both were interested in the pursuit of knowledge and in preserving the human qualities of man, and today anthropologists and nurses alike are faced with the challenge of exploring the present and potential relationships between the fields of anthropology and nursing. They are confronted with crucial questions such as: 1) What are the present and potential relationships between the fields of anthropology and nursing? 2) Is there a reciprocal contribution? 3) If so, what are the common ties between these two fields? 4) What are the mutual theoretical and research interests of members of the two fields?

Since anthropology is the field which is concerned with the holistic and generalized aspects of man, it can contribute fresh knowledge and different views of man's behavior to the field of nursing. Such knowledge can be valuable to nurses in their need to understand man's behavior from a broad cross-cultural viewpoint. One of the first and most important contributions of anthropology to nursing is the concept of *man's existence and development from a longitudinal perspective.* Realizing that man's evolutionary development began more than one million years ago and continues in the present, makes us appreciate the uniqueness of the human creature for no other mammal has had such a survival record. *Homo sapiens* is a rugged and special being who has proved himself capable of survival under a variety of adverse and precarious situations; he has learned through the course of time how to protect himself, how to withstand external threats and pressures, and how to live in relative harmony with his environment. These are a few of the key reasons why man still exists today and has not become an extinct species—a thought to appreciate man's place in the world today.

One might say that the anthropology of nursing is an attempt to understand and know man as an evolutionary being, a cultural transmitter, a protector of his own existence, and a being who has been capable of survival for many millenia. These concepts help the nurse realize man's general tendencies to protect himself under adverse circumstances, to care for himself, and to withstand external and internal species stresses. Such important anthropological findings should not only make the nurse appreciate man's longitudinal development, but also provide her with knowledge about his potential ability to maintain his health in order to survive and live effectively in his environment. To know man in his early existence living as a paleolithic cave dweller in a harsh and special kind of environment, and then to know man today living in an urban skyscraper makes one realize human life ways.

As one views man from a longitudinal perspective, one cannot help but wonder where man is going in the next million years. What will he be doing in the future? How will he be living? What new ways will he have learned to protect himself and maintain his health? How will his environment help or hinder his health state? These are some of the kinds of questions for which health personnel need to seek answers with anthropologists. Although man is a very special being, there are some reasons for realistic concern about his future existence, particularly in regard to his ability to withstand and protect himself from the consequences of modern technology and environmental changes. Some of man's technological achievements have become real threats to his continued survival.

To nursing, anthropology can contribute anthropological findings regarding man's remote and current past and his ability to adapt to a variety of life problems and situations. Man has to date successfully achieved biological, psychological, and sociocultural adaptations to many different ecological and cultural settings. Studies from the field of physical anthropology offer insights into the direction of man's skeletal development, his general physical growth and development, his genetic and structural features, and his changes in biological development. Many of these findings have relevance to nursing, as nurses seek to understand man's current and long-ranged growth and developmental health tendencies. Another interesting finding from physical anthropology is that the size of the human brain has increased considerably during man's evolutionary development, and yet the size of the female pelvis has not increased at the same growth rate. This finding is of special interest to nurses interested in the maternal and child aspects of health. What will happen to mothers and infants because of this evolutionary development? What are the adaptation abilities of mothers and infants to this finding?

A second valuable contribution of anthropology to nursing is its *cross-cultural and comparative perspective of man*. Studies of peoples from many different parts of the world provide fascinating data and help nurses understand the similarities and differences between people. Anthropologists have long used the comparative cross-cultural method to study people and to derive hypotheses and theoretical ideas about man in general. In the study of peoples in the world, they have discovered groups which are highly unique in their patterns of living, and they have also found cultures which tend to be similar to others. Usually the approach is to view each culture as a relatively unique one until findings reveal facts to the contrary. It is the cross-cultural approach which helps the scientist to be alert to not only the similarities and differences between cultures, but also to the reasons why these cultures differ in the ways that they do. This approach provides data for the scientist to test a wide range of theories about man's behavior many of which have remained unchallenged for some time. Anthropology is the discipline which has developed and consistently uses the cross-cultural approach to study and understand people.

The cross-cultural approach also provides a broad comparative picture of human nature and human behavior, and prevents scientists from becoming unduly ethnocentric. *Ethnocentrism*, a term which refers to the belief that one's own way of living, acting, and existing is the best (or preferred) way to live, tends to dominate Western man's thinking, and can greatly interfere with the validity of his knowledge about other peoples. An ethnocentric person tends to defend and protect his views without objectively looking at another person's way of thinking or behaving. From the mass of anthropological cross-cultural studies, it has become general knowledge that peoples throughout the world differ in varying ways and that the reasons why they differ are related to special factors found in each culture. It is usually difficult for an anthropologist to remain ethnocentric once he has been exposed to a wide range of data about a particular culture. It is even more difficult to remain ethnocentric if one has lived with a foreign cultural group for a period of time. Thus, the comparative approach to the study of human cultures forces the scientist to be as objective as possible and to look for factors contributing to the similarities and differences among men. It enables him to postulate generalizations from his freshly collected empirical data, and to formulate theories about the nature of man.

There is a real need for nurses to use the anthropological cross-cultural approach, not only in order to understand people as fully as possible, but more importantly to stimulate the development of cross-cultural nursing theories and techniques. Nurses need to become knowledgeable about people from other cultures and to systematically study their health practices so that they can make specific nursing care plans which are in accord with a patient's (client's) own health needs. Cross-cultural research studies in nursing are virtually non-existent; yet they would be extremely helpful to our understanding of national and international nursing practices. Although we continue to care for people from different cultural backgrounds, our knowledge of these people is often very meager. Moreover, there is a need to identify those cross-cultural concepts, theories, and principles of nursing which are universal (world-wide) in contradistinction to those which are particularistic (local or national). Currently, most nursing concepts and practices are based upon our American middle-class norms, values, and actions, and involve only limited consideration of other social classes and cultural group norms. As nurses become more aware and sensitive to other groups, they will soon discover that many of our nursing practices may not be meaningful and helpful to members of cultural groups whose norms are different. Thus, there is not only a need for a comparative approach to the study of different cultures, but also a need for cross-cultural studies of nursing practice. The present perspective on human behavior and nursing practice should be greatly modified, extended, and refined to include a wide range of different behaviors so that the nurse would extend her thinking from local middle-class health problems to world-wide cultural health problems and needs. To date, there are very few comparative nursing studies of different cultural groups with no explicit theories to examine cross-cultural nursing practices. The author believes that nurse-anthropologists should assume an active leadership role to initiate cross-cultural nursing studies. As nursing continues to move toward the development of a science of nursing, hopefully cross-cultural nursing practices and findings will be a part of this body of knowledge.

The third major contribution of anthropology to nursing is the *culture concept*. This concept will be explored more fully in chapter 4; however, a few introductory comments will be made here. *Culture* is a central and enormously important concept in anthropology; it refers to the *totality of all the learned and transmitted behaviors of a particular group of people.* With a knowledge and appreciation of the culture concept, the nurse can become more sensitive to the differences in responses of patients. For example, instead of referring to a person with a cholestectomy, in bed 200 or Ward A, the nurse who uses the cultural approach to behavior thinks of the patient as part of a particular cultural group he has been living with over a span of time. The patient's cultural background alerts the nurse to a range of possible health problems and the ways a patient's health problems may be culturally expressed. In chapters 7, 8, and 9 several nurse-patient studies are presented which reveal how cultural factors influence patients' behavior and necessitate *cultural-specific* nursing care plans and responses. The culture aspect of behavior is as crucial in the treatment of a patient as the physical and psychological aspects of his illness. The culture concept can help nurses to understand broad patterns of human behavior as well as highly specialized behavior modalities, and it can help them understand why behavior which is culturally learned and transmitted from one generation to the next is often difficult to change. With today's concern about fair treament of minority group members, it is imperative that nurses be aware of the culture concept and adjust their nursing care accordingly.

The fourth contribution of anthropology to nursing is the use of the *holistic and cultural context approach in the understanding of man.* The holistic anthropological approach emphasizes the total response of man to multiple forces in his culture. The cultural context approach advances this holistic idea with the view that the behavior of man must also be *understood within the specific and total context of man's* physical and cultural environment. Man interacts, reacts, and relates to multiple forces in his cultural, social, and physical environments, and these major variables influence greatly his behavior, perceptions, and life goals. Anthropology is the only field which endeavors to study the wholeness of man and his behavior within the total context of his daily living experiences and physical environment. This cultural context approach to the study of man helps the anthropologist to understand the natural, recurrent, and spontaneous aspects about man's daily living patterns—disclosing his adaptation abilities, social relations, and personality dispositions.

The nursing profession has long supported the concept of comprehensive patient care in which the idea of providing total nursing care needs of patients is considered as one helps a patient or client. Comprehensive care emphasizes that the patient is a total functioning person who must be recognized as an individual with special needs and problems. Thus, the cultural approach of looking at man as a person functioning in the total context of his physical and cultural environment is most compatible with the concept of comprehensive nursing care. One might say, however, that the cultural context approach provides a still broader conceptualization of the multiple dynamic forces influencing a man's behavior in a given context, more than is currently being perceived by most nurses who espouse to the concept of comprehensive patient care. The context of comprehensive nursing care is frequently viewed as the hospital nursing staff context; whereas the cultural context approach encompasses the patient's cultural setting, social relations, and the physical environment in which he lives or works each day or while he is ill.

As the nurse works with a patient (client), she should try to create a familiar sociocultural and psychological "reality" for the patient and his family in order to help the patient link his care and treatment with the realities of his on-going daily life situation. In a way, the cultural context approach to the study of man is somewhat akin to the existential approach, in that one must discover man's real being and world and let him deal with his problems and needs in his own special life context. The anthropological approach, however, differs slightly from the existential approach in that man, his cultural and physical environment are emphasized more than man's highly individualized "being" responses and problems. Sometimes nurses have only the opportunity to observe the patient in the hospital setting; whereas, observing the patient in his home environment provides new insights about the patient's culture which were never expected in the hospital setting.

The fifth anthropological contribution to nursing is *the realization that health and illness states are strongly influenced and often primarily determined by the cultural background of an individual.* Anthropologically speaking, health and illness cannot be arbitrarily separated, let alone removed, from the individual's culture. Rather, health and illness are an integral part of any cultural system, and the meaning of health and illness is derived largely from the patient's culture. All too frequently, health personnel who have only limited understanding of the meaning and significance of the culture concept may ruthlessly dissect the patient's illness from his culture. Evidence of this practice can be found when care and treatment plans are devoid of cultural data. From an anthropological viewpoint, health-illness behavior is closely linked to cultural, ecological, political, economic, religious, social, and kinship factors. Examples of this concept will be offered in Chapters 7, 8, 9 and 10 of this book. In light of current developments in our society, it is timely and important that nurses begin to focus more specifically than they have in the past on how illness and health are *cultural expressions,* and *on how cultural factors must be considered in the helping care process to people.*

The sixth important contribution of anthropology to nursing is the *cross-cultural anthropological insights into child-rearing and socialization processes of cultural groups.* Social and cultural anthropologists have been actively involved in studying the socialization processes and specific child-rearing features of different cultures. Since Margaret Mead's early work in Samoa in the late 1920's child-rearing variables such as aggression, indulgence, dependence, independence, sexual behavior, toilet training, and the oral needs of children have been studied with several cultural groups. In addition, there have been many ethnographies which have described and discussed the socialization practices of various cultural groups—that is, how socialization agents influence a child's movement into adulthood. During the past three years, the author has taught a course entitled, "Childhood and Culture" from a crosscultural stance, and students of nursing have experienced "culture shock" to learn the many different ways that children are raised around the world. After these students had acknowledged some of their ethnocentric biases, they gradually became appreciative of how different cultures tailored their child rearing practices to train a child to become an accepted and functioning member of their society. Most important, these students discovered that most cultures have unique socialization techniques and methods to help children become responsible, interested, and active participants in their culture. The nursing students were challenged to think anew about our own socialization practices, their consequences for adult behavior and how they compared with non-Western cultures. After the students had critically examined the child-rearing practices of approximately ten different cultures, they became empathetic to other kinds of child-rearing practices and began to identify the reasons why socialization agents supported the practices they did and how these practices and beliefs were closely interwoven with other facets of the culture. A number of students commented later, "It all makes sense now, for child-rearing practices are culturally defined and are closely related to the cultural practices of the people." And finally, the students discovered that in some socieites the child-rearing practices are better suited to their societal goals and culture practices (and produce less conflict) than some of our child-rearing practices.

To date, most of our child-rearing nursing concepts are based upon Anglo-American middle-class professional norms. Since many nurses are vitally interested in child-rearing, human development, and socialization processes, anthropological child-rearing studies could deepen and extend our current nursing practices and concepts. Exposure to cross-cultural study has the potential of generating new theories about child development and to question many concepts we hold dear in the teaching and practice of child care. It is reasonable to predict that child nurse researchers and clinicians will become excited about the growing anthropological knowledge in this area and will find ethnographic studies of child-rearing refreshing and stimulating. With the present request for nurses to become involved in international maternal and child health nursing programs, anthropological data about child-rearing practices will be essential for effective and successful work with people in foreign countries.

The seventh contribution of anthropology to nursing is the *participant observation field-study method.* Participant observation refers to the anthropological method in which a person in the primary role of observing people participates casually and usually directly in the daily life activities of the people being studied. The individual in this role carefully observes the social interactional patterns of the people, listens attentively to what is said (or not said), discusses his observations with the people, and observes as much of the on-going life events of the people as is possible. As Pearsall states, "The investigator chooses from the several versions of the master role: (1) complete observer; (2) observer-as-participant; (3) participant-as-observer; or (4) complete participant."[1] The goal of participant observation is to obtain the maximum possible knowledge of the people, relating to their beliefs, values, and behavior in their familiar cultural setting. This is an invaluable method for examining the meaning of behavior in context, and it provides an opportunity to check and recheck one's observations and experiences with the people. Probably no research method to date offers such complete and valid data about people. As Becker and Geer state,

"The most complete form of the sociological datum, after all, is the form in which the participant observer gathers it: An observation of some social event, the events which precede and follow it, the explanations of its meaning by participants and spectators, before, during, and after its occurrence. Such a datum gives us more information about the event under study than data gathered by any other sociological method."[2]

The participant observation method, which originated with anthropologists, has gained rapidly in use by other social scientists. The method developed as a natural, practical, and valid way of studying people. Interestingly, it is generally accepted and liked by the people under study because the researcher tries to blend in with the group as much as possible, without forcing himself on the group.

Much could be written about the strengths and limitations of the participant observation method; but, there are other published articles which offer excellent summaries on this topic.[3,4] It is the author's belief that the participant observation field-study method is a natural and potentially useful research method for nurses. To some extent, the nurse already uses this method as natural role behavior in her clinical work with people, whether in an institutional, home, or community agency. The nurse is placed in the midst of established physical, sociocultural, and psychological situations, and she is expected to observe people therein and to interact as spontaneously as possible with them. When she is involved in close interpersonal relationships with patients, the nurse tries to study the emotional, physical, and cognitive aspects of their behavior. Affective and cognitive involvement is an important function of the participant observer, and the nurse is aware of how frequently she experiences this kind of involvement. However, as she uses the participant-observation method, she must consciously recognize her biases, personal and social conflicts, and any distortion tendencies in reporting behavior.

The person who uses the participant observation method must be fully aware of the limitations, strengths, techniques, and research findings related to the method. Also important is his recognition of any major emphasis he might be giving to his role so that this emphasis is reported in his work to understand the findings. For example, he may be more of an observer than a participant, or vice versa. There are also various demands placed upon the person who uses this method, in that he may periodically feel forced to withdraw because of the physical, psychological, social, and cultural demands made on him as a participant observer. Such factors as these must be known to the nurse, who is interested in using this method. The records of anthropologists using this method can also contribute to her full utilization of the method in her professional work.

There is a pressing need for nurses to systematically and carefully study the daily lives of healthy and sick individuals. To date, there are only a few reported nursing studies in which systematic participant observations or ethnographic accounts have been compiled on health-illness behavior. The author has used the participant observation method in a psychiatric nursing and community health study of cultural groups in both urban and rural settings, and found the method to be extremely valuable in gaining rich and diversified knowledge about the day-to-day living activities of people. Indeed, the method is valuable in studying overt and covert behavior cues, in eliciting information about a specific health problem, and in checking one's suppositions about behavior with on-going participant-observations of people in their daily settings. In general, the participant-observation method can be used as a prototype for obtaining ethnographic nursing studies. It has great potential for nurse researchers and clinicians; but the nurse will first need to study the method, the role taken by the observer, the limitations and strengths of the method, and ways to collect and analyze the data obtained.

The eighth contribution of anthropology to nursing is *linguistic knowl-*

edge about comparative and descriptive language forms and their meanings. The way people from different cultural backgrounds use words, vocal utterances, gestures, and language symbols would be of much interest to nurses working with patients. Man's early use of language assumed a variety of different forms, characteristics, and meaning modalities in various parts of the world. Present-day languages are the products of language development and change over more than a million years.[5] Through the years, all cultures have changed their language forms or have made new additions to their language. In addition, some languages which existed years ago are now extinct. Anthropologists and linguists have been studying language sounds (phonetics), grammar forms (linguistic morphology), morphemes (the minimal units of distinguishable meaning), and language syntax for a number of years. They have also studied the relationship of language to culture, personality, and race. Consequently, the field of linguistic anthropology has become a highly scientific field offering many new research findings and numerous excellent methods of studying languages.

From linguistic anthropology studies, we know that culture influences the vocabulary, grammar, and phonetics of a language group. Culture has had a profound impact upon language use, change, and development. Some of the non-Western peoples have some of the most complex languages of the world, and so one cannot say that literate peoples with advanced technology have the most complex languages. Studies have also revealed that each cultural group's language incorporates only a small portion of all the possible available sounds, morphemes, and grammatical features of man's total language potential; selectivity is involved in language formation. In general, ancestral languages which refers to forms of communication before any written records were available are most interesting and informative data about man. Language makes possible the accumulation and transmital of learned behavior which is referred to as culture. Currently, one of the major differences in language between man and animal species is that human language reveals much symbolic behavioral expression whose complex forms and meanings men are continually trying to understand.

There are also many non-language forms of communication, such as sending flowers to a loved one or responding to traffic lights, which have high symbolic significance. Non-language symbols or signs (gestures, idioms, etc.) are a growing area of study which has much relevance to nursing practice. Birdwhistell, a cultural anthropologist who was instrumental in initiating the scientific study of body communication called *kinesics*, has much to offer nursing about this important branch of language and communication systems.[6]

The substantive knowledge and research methods in the field of linguistic anthropology are highly relevant to the practice of nursing and to the development of theories about communicating with patients and people in general. Nursing deals intimately with the patient's language; nurses, however, often do not recognize the meaning of symbolic expressions, and the meaning or significance of voice inflections, pitch, and gestures. It is the author's belief that once the field of kinesics is studied and understood by nurses many intriguing research projects will emerge. The use of gestural communication with sick persons has barely been tapped and is a fertile area for nursing study. General knowledge of different language expressions of cultural groups will enhance the nurse's cue response and communication with patients; in fact, the crux of therapeutic work with patients and families is dependent upon the nurse's sensitivity to linguistic expressions and upon her ability to communicate effectively.

Although other special areas of potential contribution of anthropology to nursing could be discussed, the above examples will suffice to highlight some of the most relevant areas of contribution. In general, most anthropological theories, concepts, and research findings about man have direct or indirect relevance to nursing. Anthropological knowledge is broad in scope but also specific in regard to the study of certain aspects of man: and so the nurse can draw upon this knowledge for both general and special understanding about man. Most nurses will find that the areas of psychological anthropology, social anthropology, cultural anthropology, physical anthropology, and linguistic anthropology are highly relevant to nursing practice.

FOOTNOTES

[1] Marion Pearsall, "Participant Observation as Role and Method in Behavioral Research," *Nursing Research*, Vol. 14, No. 1, Winter 1965, p. 37.

[2] Howard S. Beeker and Blanche Geer, "Participant Observation and Interviewing: A Comparison," *Human Organization*, Vol. 16, Fall 1957, p. 28.

[3] Pearsall, *op. cit.*, pp. 37-42.

[4] Elizabeth Lee Byerly, "The Nurse Researcher as Participant-Observer in a Nursing Setting," *Nursing Research*, Vol. 18, No. 3, May-June 1969, pp. 230-236.

[5] Joseph H. Greenberg, "Language and Evolution," *Man in Adaptation: The Cultural Present*, Edited by Yehudi A. Cohen, Chicago: Aldine Publishing Company, p. 39.

[6] Ray L. Birdwhistell, *Introduction to Kinesics*, Foreign Service Institute, Louisville: University of Louisville Press, 1952.

3 The Nature of Nursing and Its Contribution To Anthropology

The Nature of Nursing: the Author's Conception

The nursing profession is going through a transition of moving from a pre-scientific phase into a theoretical and scientific one; consequently, there are many changes in thinking and practice arising within the field, as well as numerous views, conflicts, and misunderstandings. In addition, the profession is facing an increase in the public demands for more and better nursing services. These developments are occurring amidst increasingly complex institutional, national, and technological problems in our society. There is also emphasis within the profession on developing truly community-centered nursing care, which has widespread implications of calling for less hospital and bureaucratic institutional modes and more community-oriented practices. These factors are reflected in the diversity of ideological health views, movements toward new programs in nursing education, and drastic changes in rendering of nursing services to people.

Since the emergence of modern nursing as a profession, much has been written in various publication outlets about nurses, nursing roles, nursing education, and nursing practice. The importance and status of nursing has been discussed along with the problems, trends, and general quality of leadership in the field. Currently, there are a variety of different philosophical, and practical views about the nature and goals of nursing, but only a few explicit formulations have been made about the nature of nursing practice. Moreover, there is no definitive or unanimous statement upon which all members of the nursing profession can agree, about *what is* or *is not* nursing. There are, however, position statements about nursing education and statements about nursing practice, plus a practice code for professional nurses. Perhaps, in the near future, some definitive statements about nursing and it's commitments to health services will be forthcoming. At this point, the author will present her own conception of and views about nursing which are based upon her work as a nurse clinician, educator, researcher, and consultant over a period of twenty-three years.

As a prefatory comment, one of the important and current problems is the conceptual and knowledge gap between the professional and average lay person's views about nursing and the nurse. Lay people, for example, generally view the nurse as a competent technician primarily at the total service of a physician and with no independent professional activities. The nurse is viewed as an extension of the physician's arms and legs. Frequently lay people do not view the nurse as a health scholar, discoverer of new knowledge, or being an independent therapist. The nurse as an "angel of mercy" is viewed as primarily responsible for the physical comfort of the "doctor's patient". Furthermore, lay people often speak of "a nurse" and seldom differentiate that there are several kinds of nurses, depending upon their educational background and professional experiences. For example, an individual who has had only six months of education may be called a "nurse" without being distinguished from the nurse who has had twelve years of rigorous professional preparation through baccalaureate, master, and doctoral programs in nursing. The resultant false expectations, frustrations, and distortions in image role are sometimes considerable. Professionally speaking, the nurse is both an independent and collaborative nurse practitioner who functions in multiple roles such as a general clinician, skilled therapist, researcher, educator, or consultant. She assumes these roles depending upon her educational preparation and experiences.

In the broadest sense, nursing refers to a body of knowledge and the specialized techniques and processes to help people with health-threatening problems or conditions. Nursing can be viewed as a helping service which is concerned with the prevention of illness and with specialized therapeutic practices to assist individuals and groups who are ill or under the threat of illness. Nursing is concerned primarily with the direct personalized care and treatment of people. The nurse, however, gives indirect nursing care to individuals and groups through her advice, guidance, and supervision of other professional nurses concerning health matters.

The author believes that the professional nurse makes one of her most significant contributions to persons through short and long-term therapeutic relationships with them. It is the therapeutic nurse-client relationship which provides largely the matrix in which specific physical, psychological, social, and cultural dimensions of care are given to people. Therapeutic nurse-client relationships are learned through our existing nursing knowledge and practices of skilled nurse clinicians in the field. In order to become a competent and effective professional nurse in dealing with complex problems and needs of people, on-going supervision is necessary to perfect and fully understand therapeutic relationship processes. In the process of helping people through therapeutic relationships, the nurse draws heavily upon interpersonal nursing knowledge and relates this knowledge to other humanistic and health science data. The nurse moves the patient toward specific health goals and deals with a variety of illness-threatening and perpetuating health problems through nurse-client relationships. Various therapeutic maneuvers and techniques of a psychological, physical and social nature are used. The nurse is especially sensitive to the oral and verbal communication expressions between the client and herself. In any therapeutic relationship the nurse's professional knowledge and skills are considered in light of the patient's cultural norms and personal strivings.

"*Care*," used as a noun, implies the provision of personalized and necessary services to help man maintain his health state or recover from an illness. "*Caring*," used as a verb, implies a feeling of compassion, interest, and concern for people. The nurse expresses her concern by providing nurturant, supportive, and succorant acts of helpfulness to her patient. The way caring is perceived, understood, and put into action by the nurse varies; however, this variability provides the necessary freedom for the nurse to blend her professional skills and knowledge with the patient and with her own philosophical and personal views about illness, health and helping man. For example, Sister Madeleine Clemence expresses beautifully the way the nurse cares for a patient on the basis of an existential philosophy.

"[The nurse who cares] does not make decisions on the patient's behalf, no matter how much wiser she may be than he in matters of health; she does not substitute her strength for the patient's weakness, not even spare him suffering at all cost. The role of the nurse is to help the patient become an authentic person and to use his situation and illness for doing so . . .

[The nurse] helps the patient to be; to be self-accepting, with insight, capable of bearing all the consequences of his actions without excuses or alibi, open to love, open to life with all its richness and diversity but also to its concomitant suffering."[1]

Nursing involves the skilled and sensitive administration of technical and non-technical aspects of therapy, together with a judicious blending of psychological, physiological, cultural, and sociological knowledge of the care-treatment process. Nursing is not the performing of tasks for other professional groups, nor acting as handmaiden to other health personnel who are not able to find time to complete their services to patients. Instead, nursing is concerned actively and vitally with all activities related to planning, coordinating, and administrating primary care to people. Finally, nursing care implies the treatment of people, in that nurses have a significant role in the healing or curing process of sick people. They are often involved in the direct administration of therapeutic aids and treatment services to patients. Of course, other members of the health professions share in the caring and treatment process, but the nurse is one of the most immediate and direct persons in initiating, coordinating, and carrying through the therapeutic care for patients.

Nurses help people through a professional relationship which is *learned*. It is the *use of a therapeutic relationship* with patients that constitutes the "heart" of nursing practice and determines what is done to the patient and how it is done. The nurse's skill in verbal and non-verbal communication, in the assessment of behavior, in making appropriate interventions, in maintaining a therapeutic relationship with patients, in the use of human and non-human community resources, and in studying health problems are essential components for a therapeutic relationship with patients. Inherent in the process of maintaining a helpful relationship with the patient, the nurse must frequently assess her own behavior and its impact upon the patient. This is important in order to maintain an on-going dynamic and therapeutic nurse-patient relationship. Supervision by skilled clinicians and teachers of nursing helps the nurse to maintain a therapeutic relationship with the patient as well as to advance her clinical competencies. Supervisory experiences are important learning experiences which keep the nurse sensitive, compassionate, and intellectually alert to the patient's needs and behavior. To become and remain an expert clinician who can deal with a variety of complex health problems requires that the nurse remain actively interested and involved in studying and dealing with nursing problems. She does this by working directly with patients, by supervisory conferences, by the use of research findings about clinical problems, and by discussing clinical problems with other nurses. The use of research findings provides the basis for modifying or reaffirming efficacious nursing practices. As a skilled clinician, the nurse is expected to identify what she did in helping the patient and to have a working knowledge of therapeutic measures she used in caring for a patient.

From a nurse-anthropologist's viewpoint, nursing is not only concerned with the above foci, but should give serious attention to *the adaptation process of man*. If nurses could focus on the *ways* in which a man adapts to his illness (physiologically, psychologically, and socio-culturally), she would have many new ideas of ways to help people. We know from anthropological data that man generally adapts to and deals with his health problems long before he sees professional health personnel, or is diagnosed as having a specific kind of illness. *Self-care adaptations are a part of man's human nature and survival.* Moreover, man tends naturally to help other sick men or those under the threat of illness. That man's illness is largely culturally and socially defined is determined by how man relates to his physical and sociocultural environments and this fact is of utmost importance to the nurse. Through time, man has developed traditional ways of adapting to illness not only for his own survival but also for the survival of his cultural group. These culturally-defined ways of adapting are often transmitted to other men in his culture and usually passed on to succeeding generations. Health and illness, then, are viewed by nurse-anthropologists primarily in terms of *culturally prescribed ways* to maintain health or to adapt to illness. In some societies illness may even be prescribed for certain social and cultural reasons. This fact may be difficult for the nurse to accept and yet can be well documented in anthropological work. As the nurse learns to take cues from the patient's cultural background, she will want to consider ways to make cultural norms a realistic part of their nursing care plans and to use cultural adaptation modalities of patients in a specific and knowledgeable way.

In general, man strives for a culturally-defined state of health—that is, one which permits him to interact with others, perform certain duties and obligations, and live in his social and cultural group without too much pain or illness. To most people, health and illness states are largely a matter of *the way one knows, sees, and understands health and illness conditions in terms of his own cultural background and perceptual screen.* This statement makes us realize that when a patient from a given cultural background interacts with a nurse from a different cultural or social orientation, he will respond to her largely in terms of his "cultural screen." Furthermore, the nurse usually discovers that many patients tend to believe that multiple forces are influencing their illness state, even though the physician may offer a single-cause of his illness. It is, therefore, important that the nurse not only use a broad cultural and social framework to understand the patient, but also to consider the patient's "cultural screen" as he views his health problems. This kind of information is essential to a therapeutic plan for the patient and to maximize the patient's ability to draw upon his own cultural resources, his own ways of interpreting his illness and helping himself get well.

Contributions of Nursing to Anthropology

There are several potential areas where nursing could make a substantial contribution to the field of anthropology. First, and most obvious, is *the nurse's personalized knowledge of people when they are ill or experiencing the threat of illness.* During the course of the nurse's interaction with the patient, she observes and identifies many intimate, personal, and recurrent tendencies of people who are ill. She discovers that man exhibits both common and highly idiosyncratic behavior when ill. For example the nurse has frequently observed that when a person becomes suddenly and acutely ill he tends to express dependence in a variety of ways, and for short or long periods of time. As Western man regains his health state, he makes decisions (largely unconscious) as to whether he will resort to dependency, become independent, or play an interdependent role—much depends upon factors in his cultural situation, his psychological tendencies, and his past experiences with illness. Dependency is a recurrent behavioral tendency of man observed by nurses in our society.

Another behavior trait observed by nurses in Western society is *the high selectivity of special human and nonhuman resources a patient will use to help him recover or remain in an illness state.* This selectivity in the use of resources and the responses of some patients to have similar kinds of illnesses is noteworthy. This behavior seems to be dependent upon Western man's socialization practices regarding health and illness. Another aspect of the nurses experience that anthropologists would find interesting is her knowledge that *extensive physical insult to the human body not only incapacitates the individual physically, but generally produces concomitant psychological and social trauma.* This fact alerts the nurse to look for psycho-physiological and social behavior responses, and not to isolate these responses from one another. Losing a body appendage, for example, generally changes a person's self-image, self-aspirations, and motivations for living: consequently, the nurse can anticipate that the patient will reveal a low self-esteem and a depressed behavioral state. The above kinds of personalized responses and general knowledge about patients provide informative data for anthropologists in their search for understanding of the broad behavioral tendencies of man. The professional nurse can provide a wealth of rich data about man's general psycho-physiological responses to illness which should be particularly useful to anthropologists in their efforts to assess man's biological and psychological adaptation abilities and to compare Western man's behavior with that of non-Western peoples. And finally as the nurse observes the patient's response to illness she is exposed to the adaptation abilities of adults and children, of males and females, and to a wide array of illness conditions. Such information could be useful to anthropologists as they seek for behavioral differences among males and females and between adults and children cross-culturally.

A *second* major contribution which nurses can make to the field of *anthropology is providing access to people for firsthand health data.* Traditionally, nurses have had an unprecedented natural entree into the sick person's hospital room, home, and into other settings where sick persons are found. No other health personnel (not even physicians) have had such a natural and generally accepted way to reach the ill. The author has frequently heard psychologists and social scientists say, "I wish I could enter the patient's room or home as easily as you nurses can. You seem to have free access." Nurses hope that people will continue to accept and trust nurses in this manner. Thus nurses can help anthropologists and others who may be having difficulty reaching people to study their health and illness patterns. Anthropologists have in the past had a fairly spontaneous entree into villages, homes and community agencies; however, where illness is involved they may encounter some difficulty because the illness may constitute a crisis in which outsiders are not wanted unless they are willing to help the patient. Cross-culturally, special health practitioners such as the shaman or the medicine men, and some professional staff have had access to the patient and his family. Thus the nurse, may be helpful in assisting anthropologists to gain access to sick people; reciprocally, anthropologists can often help nurses get into "well" homes and community agencies through their field study methods, expertise, and general acceptance by people in a given community. Recently the author was functioning in the role of an anthropologist as she studied a Spanish-American community and nurses were assisting with the study of "well" families. Some of these families were quite reluctant to let a nurse enter their homes, since their traditional view of nurses was that they were only concerned with sickness problems. The anthropologist was able to help the nurses gain entry into the home since the families had developed considerable mutual trust and respect for her.

The third contribution the nurse can make to anthropology is *information about the wide range of actual and potential health problems and circumstances which individuals and families experience.* As the nurse moves from one situation, event, or crisis setting to another, she observes the variety of health problems that people experience in an array of different circumstances. Although the nurse has not systematically documented these phenomena, she is generally able to describe and compare these varying circumstances and the health problems manifest in each setting. These data would be fascinating for anthropological investigation, particularly in determining man's scope of illness response in multiple kinds of settings and environments. A collaborative research study could be planned with special contributions from the nurse and the anthropologist.

A fourth contribution is what the author calls *the "self-other awareness" method* used in nursing practice. One of the crucial methods of helping people, which has been particularly developed and used in psychiatric nursing practice, is self-awareness and understanding of one's own behavior in relation to others. Therapeutic nursing practice is predicated upon this belief that long-range and effective care is possible only as a consequence of this essential nursing ingredient. Nurses are being taught to be cognizant of their own behavior and the behavior of others in short-term and in long-term relationships. Being cognizant of one's own feelings, attitudes, and actions is crucial in finding effective means of helping others. Process recordings, clinical logs, and supervision from skilled nurse therapists are some of the common methods utilized in nursing to maintain a high degree of self-other awareness behavior. These methods aim to make the nurse as objective and knowing about her behavior as possible in relation to different people and situations.

Although the need for self-other awareness is known to anthropologists, still there is a need to make the anthropologist more sensitive and fully cognizant of his own behavioral tendencies and their impact upon other people. Social scientists and professional workers need to give serious consideration to this aspect of their work. Hallowell,[2] Bohannon,[3] Malinowski,[4] and others have clearly recognized the importance of self-objectivity in field work. More direct and conscious efforts, however, are needed to help anthropologists recognize how their own behavior influences people's responses and thus influences their own research findings. Some of the nursing methods mentioned above such as, the use of process recordings and daily observation logs could be used by anthropologists to increase their sensitivity to people and to note their own behavioral tendencies. In addition, it is the author's view that more emphasis should be given by teachers of anthropology to self-other awareness behavior especially in field method courses. Although psychological anthropologists have recognized the importance of behavior and the impact of the anthropologist upon the cultural group he is studying, still the methods and process to help field anthropologists understand and deal with this problem have been limitedly handled. In a recent article Osborne, a nurse-anthropologist, recognizes the potential value of anthropologists using nursing methods related to self-knowledge and self-understanding.[5]

A fifth potential contribution which the nurse can make to anthropology is *information about the verbal and nonverbal patterns of communication people adopt as they move from a wellness to a sickness role and vice versa.* The nurse generally has excellent opportunities to obtain knowledge about such behavior. Unfortunately, this area of study and knowledge is not fully recognized or developed by nurses. Nonetheless the potential for making a substantial contribution to the field of anthropology is considerable. Questions such as the following could be systematically studied: How does man tend to modify his communication patterns when he becomes ill? How is illness behavior expressed through nonverbal forms of communication? What is the range of this behavior? What is the function of changes in verbal and nonverbal communication when people move from a wellness to a sickness role? Linguistic anthropologists could collaborate with nurses on the study of these significant questions. It is the author's theory that individuals who are ill tend to use more nonverbal forms of communication than verbal; in fact, gestural and other forms of nonverbal communication are extremely important as sources of knowledge in understanding illness behavior. Nurses also receive messages which linguistic anthropologists might be able to decode and structurally analyze more accurately than nurses.

In their socialization process, nurses learn to become sensitive to gestural cues and other forms of nonverbal communication, and they base their assessment of a child's or an adult's health status upon many nonverbal cues. These gestural cues and their meanings, however, could be made explicit and should be documented. Nurses could use the ethnoscientific method of anthropology to scientifically study and report the gestural communication forms of sick persons (see Chapter 11). Multiple forms of gestural behavior related to pain, suffering, and illness expressions which have cultural meaning are just beginning to be studied. In general, the nurse is in a strategic position to help with the documentation of gestural sickness behavior and to make inferences about the meaning of this behavior.

Finally, and perhaps most importantly, *the nurse can contribute her own personal experiences and philosophical views about the care and treatment of people and about sick behavior as a common and recurrent human phenomena.* Ethnographic studies of the nursing care of people would offer valuable knowledge about man's needs for care and about man's behavior, as well as about the process of getting well and becoming ill. Currently, we have no ethnographic accounts of man's actual sick role behavior with related nursing care practices. Nor do we have documental accounts of man's basic care needs and interest in caring for others. There are, however, some studies which have been made by ethologists on care process and nurturant responses in sub-human species. Since care is an important component of nursing, one wonders how important care has been and is today for man's survival. What is the cultural variability of man's responses to care as concern for others? To nurturance as growth maintenance? To succorance as dependent support to another person? Is care a quality unique to *homo sapiens*? Does man thrive on giving care and receiving care? These questions and others make us pause to consider how much we have yet to learn about concepts related to care and caring and their variability among people of other countries.

Other potential areas in which the nurse can make a contribution to anthropology will unfold as nurses become more oriented and knowledgeable about the field of anthropology. Some of the areas which were not discussed in this chapter are social system behavior in institutions, patterns of communication in health systems, social and political systems affecting nursing care practices, role socialization in nursing, and international health-illness practices. Anthropological insights about people could be valuable to nurses in developing community nursing programs and in gaining a broad understanding of people. There are many rich and exciting possibilities for collaborative work between anthropologists and nurses; indeed, the future looks most promising if rapprochement of the two fields is to occur.

Facts and Hunches About the Delayed Interest of Nursing in Anthropology

Although nursing and anthropology have similar birthdates, the bond of interest between the two fields has been weak and slow to develop. In this section an exploration will be made of some of the possible reasons why anthropological concepts have not yet become an integral part of nursing.

It is well known that the practice of nursing has traditionally focused primarily upon the physiological and psychological health needs of man, while only a tacit acknowledgement has been made of man's social needs. Even today, nurses are held responsible on state board and national examinations primarily for physiological and psychological principles and concepts. Very few items on these exams are sociological or culturological. Currently and in the past, nurses have not been expected to understand the cultural dimensions of health. The three traditional areas have provided only a partial picture to understand the basis of man's health behavior, as the cultural dimension to health is missing and needs to become an integral part of nursing thought and practice.

One of the major reasons why cultural aspects have not been a part of the nurse's thinking is that the nurse in her educational preparation has not been sufficiently exposed to the field of anthropology. Currently, anthropology courses are not required, nor even recommended as electives in most basic nursing programs. Nursing students are explicitly required today to take courses such as anatomy, physiology, chemistry, sociology, psychology, and nursing, together with some courses in the humanities. In 1968, the author conducted a survey to determine the comparative offerings in schools of nursing of anthropology, sociology, and psychology courses. The findings revealed that of the surveyed National League for Nursing accredited undergraduate schools of nursing, less than one per cent required anthropology courses, and only ten per cent offered anthropology courses as electives.[6] Table I reveals the total number of social science (anthropology, psychology, and sociology) courses offered by ninety-one NLN accredited baccalaureate schools of nursing in the United States in 1968.

One can note the marked emphasis upon psychology and sociology courses and the limited emphasis upon required and elective courses in anthropology. These findings were comparable to those found in the graduate nursing programs in the United States. (The detailed findings of this study will be reported in the near future.) Perhaps part of the problem may be related to the fact that nursing faculty who have never had a course in anthropology find it difficult to appreciate and understand the contribution which anthropology can make to nursing. Hopefully, there will be more faculty interested in increasing anthropological content in nursing programs.

TABLE I
TOTAL REQUIRED AND ELECTIVE SOCIAL SCIENCE COURSES IN NINETY-ONE UNDERGRADUATE NURSING PROGRAMS

Fields	Required	(Mean)	Electives	(Mean)
Anthropology	17	.18	23	.25
Psychology	176	2.92	43	.47
Sociology	142	1.56	58	.63

Total Number of Courses and Mean

The field of medicine began to show an interest in anthropology during the 1920's. Several physicians (primarily psychiatrists) collaborated with anthropologists to study the relations between culture and personality, and the physical anthropological aspects of man. A survey by the author in 1968 revealed that there were approximately 370 published articles in medical and anthropological literature and five books dealing specifically with anthropology and medicine. These figures are in contrast with developments in the field of nursing. To date (July, 1969), there are only nineteen published articles dealing with anthropology and nursing, and there are no books which focus specifically upon nursing in relation to anthropology. Furthermore, there has been some difficulty getting articles accepted for publication by qualified nurse-anthropologists in nursing journals. The material has been declined because the "material does not seem to be relevant to nursing."

Several well-known anthropologists have been interested in the field of nursing, and have contributed their knowledge and special insights from an anthropological viewpoint about patient care problems, milieu therapy, social structure features, and cultural norms of institutions, patients, and nurses. Two cultural anthropologists, Esther Lucille Brown and Ray Birdwhistell, were early contributors and have remained actively interested in the interrelationship of anthropology and nursing. In 1949, Birdwhistell addressed the National League for Nursing and identified several areas where anthropological insights would be useful to nurses.[7] In this paper, he discussed how differences in the social class and cultural background of patients and nurses influenced the expectations that each held of the other. Esther Lucille Brown became well known in the field of nursing, beginning with her early publication, *Nursing as a Profession*, published in 1936.[8] *Nursing for the Future*, published in 1948, offered insight into nursing and its future directions.[9] She also wrote some articles regarding the use of social science concepts in nursing to improve patient care. In 1961,[10] 1962,[11] and 1964,[12] she contributed a series of monographs on the theme "Newer Dimensions of Patient Care." Her body of work has been sizeable and invaluable in helping nurses to take a fresh look at nursing practices and in suggesting guidelines for the future of nursing education and practice.

A number of other well-known anthropologists have also been active contributors to the field of nursing, including Margaret Mead, William Caudill, Otto Von Mering, Lyle Saunders, Solon Kimball, and others. Their research studies and/or publications regarding cultural factors influencing patient needs and the treatment and care problems of patients from an anthropological perspective have been extremely helpful in considering new modalities in working with patients as people. Saunders' article (1954) was important in helping nurses understand the changing role of the nurse in our culture and her future role in patient care.[13]

Interestingly, the first article which focused upon cultural factors and patient care was written by a nurse and was written in 1960.[14] McCabe wrote how the hospital patient care would be improved if social and cultural factors of patients were taken into account. Since 1965, there has been a small core of professional nurse-anthropologists in the United States who have completed doctoral programs in anthropology, and these nurses are contributing in various ways to nursing by their teaching, writing, research, and clinical work.[15] Undoubtedly, these nurses and others completing a similar program of study will be a significant force in bringing anthropology and nursing closer together.

In 1965, Jacobs presented an interesting paper on the status of medical personnel in relation to using anthropologists and anthropological insights in patient care. She identified several reasons why anthropological knowledge was not an integral part of patient care.[16]

The author has given further thought to the problem of why anthropology has not become an integral part of nursing and has identified several reasons. First, from a historical viewpoint, nursing has been affected by societal and cultural forces which have influenced the direction of its development. As one looks at the evolution of nursing, one finds that during the early Christian era, nursing was in the hands of notable women who were devoted to caring for the physical needs of people. It was not until the middle of the nineteenth century that Florence Nightingale, the founder of professional nursing, saw the need to raise the social status of nursing by making it a respectable, knowledgeable, and disciplined field. The ardent, assiduous, and lengthy struggle to educate women as professional nurses was Florence Nightingale's commendable goal. Her philosophical view of nursing as a field in which both knowledge and integrity were important influenced the development of the profession. During this early nursing period, crisis situations and the sheer meeting of humanitarian physical and some social needs of ill people did not permit the nurse to consider or even speculate about man's universal and cultural health needs. At that time the field of anthropology was also in its infancy so that there was only limited knowledge upon which nurses could draw to help them understand man in a broad perspective. After the turn of the twentieth century, the scientific medical era occurred and there was marked emphasis upon surgery, asepsis, medicine, diseases, and contagion. The nurse was literally swept into this trend and was preoccupied with maintaining asepsis, administering medications and a variety of treatments, and sundry administrative tasks necessary to assure that the surgical and medical needs of patients would be supported. As a consequence, nursing became noticeably engulfed in the physical and biological dimensions of patient care, and nurses found only limited opportunity to consider the social, psychological, and cultural needs of patients.

During World War II, the nurse was gradually exposed to the psychological and psychosomatic aspects of patient care and treatment. This development soon led to a heightened interest in the Freudian and Neo-Freudian psychodynamic approach to understanding patient behavior. Psychiatric nursing took the leadership in incorporating psychological aspects into the nursing care of patients. Although a few psychiatrists and physicians were using anthropological concepts in patient care, nursing remained oblivious to the content and findings of anthropology. Nursing did, however, begin to talk about the social aspects of patient care. (It is a point worth noting that Nightingale herself mentioned the "social needs" of patients.) But the meaning and significance of social aspects of patient care were only limitedly understood by nurses since their educational program provided practically none of the knowledge necessary to understand human social needs. Only recently, with the growing number of nurse sociologists with doctoral preparation in sociology, are nurses beginning to understand the sociological concepts useful to nursing practice. In a similar evolution, cultural factors related to patient care are just beginning to be understood. The latest cliche in nursing is to speak of the "bio-psycho-social" needs of man. The cultural dimension is omitted and, consequently these needs are not emphasized.

From this brief historical sketch, one begins to realize what was emphasized at different periods in the history of nursing. Certainly, the cultural aspects have not been a part of the nurse's thinking and way of helping patients until very recently.

Another reason why nursing practice has been slow to integrate anthropology is that there is a very limited number of nurse-anthropology role models in nursing; there are only a handful of nurse-anthropologists teaching in nursing schools and in hospital and community settings. Thus the professional nurse and the nursing student have only a meager opportunity to observe and gain knowledge from a nurse-anthropologist. Because of this fact, nurses have had a difficult time understanding how anthropology can become a part of the nurse's mode of thinking and acting.

Statistics reveal that there are only a few nurse-anthropologists and anthropologists employed in schools of nursing. From the author's study in 1968, there were only eight full-time anthropologists (four in undergraduate programs and four in the graduate programs) and no part-time anthropologists in ninety-one schools of nursing having graduate and undergraduate units of instruction.[17]

Table II shows where the emphasis is in nursing education and the ratio of anthropologists to sociologists and psychologists in schools of nursing.

Jacobs made a survey of twenty-five major hospitals associated with medical or nursing schools, and revealed that there were no anthropologists employed in these hospitals.[18] She had received a 100 per cent reply. Hopefully, more anthropologists will soon be employed in schools of nursing, medicine, and dentistry as well as in hospital and community health agencies. Because of the limited number of anthropologists in health centers, it will be a while before the staff can recognize their special and unique contribution. Psychiatric personnel seem quite interested in and receptive to the role of an anthropologist on a psychiatric team. They have also used anthropologists as consultants, more so than other professional health personnel. This has been because psychiatry encounters directly expressions of behavior which are culturally derived. It has been the author's experience that psychiatric staff have been stimulated by anthropological insights and have endeavored to apply such knowledge to the patient treatment plan. In addition, some fruitful research areas combining psychiatry and anthropology have been uncovered.

TABLE II
FULL-TIME AND PART-TIME SOCIAL SCIENTISTS EMPLOYED IN NINETY-ONE NLN ACCREDITED SCHOOLS OF NURSING IN SEPTEMBER, 1968

Social Scientists and Program	Full-Time	Part-Time	Number of Schools
Anthropologists			
Undergraduate	4	0	60
Graduate	4	0	31
Total	8	0	91
Psychologists			
Undergraduate	7	0	60
Graduate	24	2	31
Total	41	2	91
Sociologists			
Undergraduate	17	0	60
Graduate	12	1	31
Total	26	2	91

In general, psychiatric personnel view the anthropologist as a helpful person to understand the cultural and social features of behavior and for suggesting how to deal with cultural behavior in the treatment of patients.

Another reason for the dormant interest of nurses in anthropology is that patients have been extremely tolerant and have not demanded that their cultural and social needs be recognized. Patients from some minority cultural backgrounds have, in the past, been rather deferent, passive, and tolerant about their cultural needs when confronted by health personnel. One might view their deferent attitude as a superordinate-subordinate response to other dominant cultural groups. As a consequence of this attitude, most minority cultural groups have not urgently requested health personnel to give more explicit attention to their culturally defined needs and problems. As a consequence, many nurses, physicians, and other health workers have been able to avoid, deny, or gloss over the cultural and social needs of patients. There is evidence, however, that patients and families are becoming more vocal than they have been in the past in regard to their cultural needs and problems. And one can anticipate that in the near future their needs will become patently known and demands will be made for attention. Already, some cultural groups have become sensitive to discriminatory practices regarding their health needs. Others have demanded that their cultural, social, and economic health problems be given as much consideration as their physical and psychological problems. The day has come when we can no longer overlook the cultural aspects of each patient's health needs. Health personnel will need to work fast in procuring knowledge that will help them deal effectively with people from different cultural backgrounds. One can anticipate that people will confront the nurse more and more with their natural right to have their cultural needs understood and met.

Finally, the reason for the late interest of nurses in anthropology is found in the nurses' conceptions and misconceptions about the field of anthropology. For the past four years, the author has taught a number of undergraduate and graduate nursing students in such courses related to health, culture, and nursing. It has been of interest to discover that more than two-thirds of the nursing students had no previous courses in anthropology. In addition, the author was interested in the students' initial ideas about anthropology, and so they were asked to write their major ideas about what they thought anthropology was. The responses disclosed that the students had only a meager grasp of the field. Their most common and recurrent responses were the following: (1) "The field is concerned with digging up ancient bones to determine something about man"; (2) "I really don't have any idea of what anthropologists do, or about the field of anthropology" (54 percent gave this response); (3) "Anthropologists are mainly interested in primitive and exotic people and how they lived"; (4) "Anthropology is interested in the peculiar customs of people in remote places in the world." As one can discern from these responses, the students were uncertain about the nature of anthropology, and most of them thought that anthropology is primarily concerned with ancient man living in remote places of the world. There were only a few students who were aware that anthropology deals with modern man and with man's behavior in our own culture as well as in Western subcultural groups. They, too, had no idea that anthropologists are concerned with social and cultural system behavior especially in hospitals and health agencies. Although the nurse's knowledge of anthropology was, at first, limited, it was gratifying to note their rapid and heightened interest as they studied anthropological content and tried to apply these ideas to nursing situations. As nurses become more exposed to anthropological ideas, it is safe to predict that there will be a satisfying and fairly rapid assimilation of these concepts into nursing practice.

FOOTNOTES

[1]Sister Madeleine Clemence Vaillot, "Existentialism: A Philosophy of Commitment," *American Journal of Nursing*, March 1966, Vol. 66, 500-505.

[2]Irving Hollowell, *Culture and Experience*, Pennsylvania: University of Pennsylvania Press, 1955.

[3]Paul Bohannon, *Social Anthropology*, New York: Holt, Rinehart, and Winston, 1963.

[4]Bronislaw Malinowski, *Argonauts of the Pacific*, New York: E. P. Dutton and Company, 1961 (paperback), pp. 1-26.

[5]Oliver H. Osborne, "Anthropology and Nursing: Some Common Traditions and Interests," *Nursing Research*, May-June, 1969. Vol. 18, No. 3, 251-255.

[6]Madeleine Leininger, "Study of Social Science Courses Taught in Baccalaureate and Graduate NLN Accredited Schools of Nursing in the United States," unpublished report, 1968.

[7]Ray L. Birdwhistell, "Social Science and Nursing Education: Some Tentative Suggestions," Fifty-Fifth Annual Report of the National League of Nursing Education, 1949, pp. 315-328.

[3]Esther Lucille Brown, *Nursing as a Profession*, New York: Russell Sage Foundation, 1936.

[9]Esther Lucille Brown, *Nursing for a Future*, New York: Russell Sage Foundation, 1948.

[10]Esther Lucille Brown, *Newer Dimensions of Patient Care, Part I: The Use of Physical and Social Environment of the General Hospital for Therapeutic Purposes*, New York: Russell Sage Foundation, 1961.

[11]Esther Lucille Brown, *Newer Dimensions of Patient Care, Part II: Improving Staff Motivation and Competence in the General Hospital*, New York: Russell Sage Foundation, 1962.

[12]Esther Lucille Brown, *Newer Dimensions of Patient Care, Part III: Patients as People*, New York: Russell Sage Foundation, 1964.

[13]Lyle Saunders, "The Changing Role of Nurses," *American Journal of Nursing*, Vol. 54, 1954, pp. 1094-98.

[14]Garcia S. McCabe, "Cultural Influences on Patient Behavior," *American Journal of Nursing*, Vol. 60, No. 8, August 1960, pp. 1101-1104.

[15]As of July 1, 1969, there were seven nurse-anthropologists who had completed a Ph.D. doctoral program in anthropology. There are, however, other nurses enrolled in doctoral programs in anthropology who have taken anthropology courses or had anthropology as part of their program of study, and these nurses are also making a contribution to the field.

[16]Sue Ellen Jacobs, "Anthropology and Nursing", unpublished paper given at the Sixty-Fourth Annual Meeting of the American Anthropological Association, Denver, Colorado, 1965.

[17]Leininger, *op cit.*

[18]Jacobs, *op. cit.*

4 The Culture Concept and American Culture Values In Nursing

More than twenty years have elapsed since Margaret Mead made this perceptive statement, but its relevance could never be more important than it is to us today:

> If we are to achieve a richer culture, rich in contrasting values, we must recognize the whole gamut of human potentialities, and so weave a less arbitrary social fabric, one in which each diverse human gift will find a fitting place.[2]

The full recognition and knowledge of cultural diversities and the essential qualities of each culture group can enrich our practice of nursing. This recognition would challenge the nurse to make her care of patients more specific, refined, and culture-focused.

The scientific and humanistic integration of culture aspects into health practices is a relatively new undertaking for health practitioners. It is, however, an extremely important part of providing for optimal care to patients. Today, more than ever before, there is a need to understand people from different cultures and to use this knowledge in the helping process. No longer can health personnel respond only to the physical and psychological needs of people, but they must become sensitive and respond to their cultural and social needs.

Patients have a *right* to have their sociocultural backgrounds understood in the same way they expect their physical and psychological needs to be recognized and understood. Professional personnel must ask themselves: What do I understand about cultural differences in patient care? How do I use this knowledge in helping people? What will be the response of patients when I use cultural data in providing for patient care?

In recent years, a few social scientists have been involved in studying how professional health practitioners affect the health programs and status of cultural groups when the indigenous health practices differ considerably from the norms of the professional group. For some time, the practice has been for Western professional groups to initiate new health programs or change indigenous non-Western practices to Western standards. By and large, these health practices have been based primarily upon the norms of the Western nursing and medical practices which often differ considerably from the health norms of local and non-Western cultures. The consequences of these well-motivated and assumed health-promoting endeavors have been generally unfavorable, in that the new health programs tend to be misunderstood by the people and tend to achieve only short-ranged success.[3] Since many of these health programs did not give careful consideration to the health norms and interests of the indigenous group, one must ask what would have happened if care and treatment had been consciously designed and implemented with thought given to the indigenous people's health norms? What benefits come from a health advocacy program? Unfortunately, many health personnel cannot deal with these questions because they do not always realize that most cultures have their own health norms and practices which have been tested and used for many years and by many different generations. Currently, we must ask ourselves these related questions: What preparation and efforts have been made by Western professional personnel to understand non-Western health practices? Once understood, how could native practices be integrated with professional health practices? Why do some cultural groups show an initial interest in modern professional health services, but later abandon these practices? These and other questions make us realize how much professional health personnel have yet to learn about different cultures and their responses to "imported" health programs. Indeed, anthropological studies about the impact and consequences of our modern health programs upon other cultures indicate the need for a comprehensive understanding of other cultural groups before the programs are introduced. Results have been particularly unsatisfactory in trying to apply Western health norms to the health norms of a non-Western society.[4,5,6]

In working with people whose cultural backgrounds differ from ours, there is a natural tendency for our ethnocentrism to emerge. Ethnocentrism occurs when we contend that our professional health practices are superior to the health norms and practices of another group; we have a built-in bias that our own ways are the best and most effective. As we become familiar with another culture, however, and learn to appreciate why certain values and norms are effective through time in that culture, we become, hopefully, less ethnocentric. Most cultures, like our own, have devised health practices which fit their own particular way of life. There is, in every culture literally, a working through, testing, and retesting of beliefs and practices so that they become recognized and acceptable to the people. Anthropological studies reveal a general tenacity of traditional health beliefs, their integration into the total way of life of the people, and their pervasive influence on the people's actions and thoughts. In general, one can assume that traditional health practices are an integral part of the total culture and are generally not easily relinquished by the members of that culture. Our efforts to effect changes in the health practices of people whose cultural backgrounds differ from ours should be accompanied by as thorough an understanding of the indigenous health beliefs as possible, and a carefully developed plan for working with the people to effect changes in their health practices.

A New Dimension for Nursing

Understanding cultural factors related to patient care is essentially a new dimension and focus for nursing. It is the author's belief that a new phase and quality of health services to people will develop as health personnel begin to fully utilize cultural and social data related to health and illness. Of special interest is the fact that in the very early era of health services, much emphasis was given to the *physical* needs of patients, with only slight recognition of their sociopsychological needs. Later (about the 1930's and 1940's), there was a heavy emphasis on recognizing the psychological needs of patients, but at the same time not neglecting their physical needs. This psychological emphasis occurred as a result of the impact of psychoanalytical thinking and psychosomatic research in the medical field. During this time, some tacit recognition was given to the "social needs of patients;" however, the social aspects of patient care were only vaguely conceived and integrated into treatment. Recently there has been a conscious and open recognition of the impact of sociocultural, economic, and political forces upon health services and patient care. With this latest awareness, we can anticipate that health personnel will be more actively involved in coping with specific problems related to these aspects of health care.

In the examination of health-related aspects, one finds there has been more attention given to social aspects of patient care than there has been to the cultural aspects. The reasons can be found and understood. To begin with, one can confidently say that anthropological concepts, theories, and findings have barely penetrated the thinking and modes of action of health personnel, and especially in nursing.[7] This is strange, since anthropology deals with the general study of man and information from this field has probably the greatest potential for understanding people who are well and ill. Only from a baseline of knowledge about man, can health personnel reasonably understand why people behave as they do and what forms of health practices will help or hinder people's well being. The author proposes that the new trend in health services to use cultural and general anthropological knowledge in the care and treatment of people will greatly enhance health care services. Moreover, with this new approach can come some imaginative and creative ways of helping people and of promoting new health care models in the delivery of health services.

The Meaning of the Culture Concept

The term "culture" is probably one of the most central, most used, and important theoretical concept in the field of anthropology. It was first conceived by anthropologists, and continues to be refined and tested by social scientists. Many books have been written about culture, and more than 250 definitions of the term have been recorded.[8] The concept of "culture" as used by anthropologists is a scientific one, and differs from the layman's use of the word. In fact, the term suffers from conceptual confusion because many people rely upon the layman's view of the concept. For the layman, "culture" may be associated with a city which has an art center, a museum, a symphony, an educational center, and other special features which maintain the city's identity as a "cultured place." The layman's conception of culture is often equivalent to the high social status of a particular group of people, a refinement in social learning, the possession of special knowledge (usually related to the fine arts), and/or the ability to display certain forms of social etiquette, as evident in one's talk or mannerisms (e.g., wearing a hat or gloves at certain social gatherings). Frequently, the use of the word "culture" in this sense implies the ability of a person who is "cultured" to manipulate certain aspects of our civilization to achieve certain desired social goals. This group of "cultured people," who generally come from the upper-middle class, constitute only a special and partial segment of our society. However, they share a number of other behavior attributes with other people in our society—often more than they wish to believe.

For the social scientist, "culture" has a specific meaning. In the broadest sense, *culture* refers to *a way of life belonging to a designated group of people.* Herskovits offers a short definition of culture as "the man-made part of the environment."[9] He has also made the following theoretical postulates about the nature of culture, which help us to understand the concept: (1) "Culture is universal in man's experience, yet each local or regional manifestation of it is unique; (2) culture is stable, yet is also dynamic, and manifests constant change; and (3) culture fills and largely determines the course of our lives, yet rarely intrudes into conscious thought."[10] Each of these seemingly paradoxical statements reveals essential attributes of the culture concept. Culture is a universal experience of mankind, yet there are no two cultures which are precisely alike. Some cultures are strikingly different from others, while between other cultures there are only slight differences. In general, one finds that wherever cultural groups exist there are similar aspects among cultures as well as aspects which differentiate one culture from another. Areas of differences and similarities exist in language, material items, religious beliefs, eating habits, social organizations, and so on. The more obvious the cultural differences are between particular cultures, the more clearly one can appreciate and understand the relevance of the concept of culture.

Culture may be viewed as a blueprint for living which guides a particular group's thoughts, actions, and sentiments. Culture is a product of man's recurrent responses to various life problems which he encounters daily throughout history. Culture provides some ready-made solutions to these life problems; however, as each cultural group is confronted with new life problems, they have to devise new solutions to them if the old solutions are not effective. Culture includes all the accumulated ways a group of people solve problems, which are reflected in the people's language, dress, food, and a number of accumulated traditions and customs. It also includes material items, and the many social institutions which embody and sustain all these elements. The *material culture* is reflected in the items which man produces as a result of his creative thinking and technology. The *non-material culture* consists of many intangible items and abstract culture expressions, such as the ideologies or beliefs embodied in social and political institutions. Culture is the means by which a man can adapt and adjust to changes in his enviroment with some feeling of security and familiarity. As White states, "the purpose and function of culture are to make life secure and enduring to the human species."[11] So culture can provide reassurance and ready-made solutions to life problems; it is valuable in safeguarding the mental, cultural, physical, and social health of human beings.

Culture is not biologically inherited; rather, it is *learned and transmitted* systematically from one generation to another, largely through socialization practices which are reinforced through cultural and social institutions. The extent to which cultural aspects are shared uniformly among the members of a culture may vary considerably. On the one hand, the extent of cultural sharing may be limited to certain persons in the culture, such as in the style of dressing. On the other hand, cultural sharing with dress styles and religious practices may be quite uniform among a cultural group. It is always of interest to observe how many persons in a culture are alike and how many differ. Similarities and differences in cultural characteristics among and between cultural groups stimulates the thinking of students to speculate upon the reasons for such occurrences.

Another important feature of the concept of culture is that it is *dynamic and changing*. Although cultural groups generally reinforce certain valued norms of people to support a way of life, culture can change its values and in a relatively short period of time. Therefore culture must not be viewed as a static concept, but rather as a dynamic, changing one. There is evidence that cultures do change, but the ways they change may vary and be unpredictable. At the same time, there are cultural groups who seem fairly static and change slowly through a period of time. Why such differences exist in the rate and kind of changes is a topic studied by cultural anthropologists.

Manifest and Ideal Culture

Culture behavior may be classified into two major categories: *manifest culture* and *ideal culture*. Manifest culture refers to the pattern of actions, beliefs, and feelings which can be readily identified by any person, since they are visible to outsiders. Manifest culture reveals what people are actually doing and saying in their daily way of living. In contrast, *ideal culture* refers to the beliefs, practices, and feelings which the people hold as desirable, although they do not always live by these norms. People may say that they do this or believe in that as something of great value to them, but as one observes and studies these people they do not actually practice what they say. For example, the Gadsup people of New Guinea, whom I lived with and studied for one year, said they were generous to all their "brothers" in the village. In reality, their generosity to their "brothers" was an ideal, for their giving was restricted to a few close kinsmen and not to all the village people whom they called "brothers." One needs to be alert to the differences between the ideal (believed-in) culture and the manifest (actually practiced) culture of any group of people.

Culture and Subculture

As indicated above, culture is defined as a way of life for a particular group of people; however, culture can also be viewed as a universal in man's experience. In other words, culture is a universal experience found among all men in all places of the world. Culture, therefore, is an abstraction of behavior which is characteristic of man in general. Members of a society may share many values, beliefs, and feelings which make them members of that particular society. For example, one may speak of "the American culture" or "the national character of the American people," and contrast the American culture with other cultures. The language, style of dress, living patterns, educational values, sentiments, occupations, and religious expressions of our American culture provide data to help identify the common attributes of our culture. This broad concept of culture gives us a general picture of what we may expect to find in our American culture. Nonetheless, there still exist variations in American behavior, with subgroups and specific individuals showing slight differences from the generalized view.

There are subgroups within our American society whose members have their *own* particular sets of cultural values, beliefs, and practices. These subgroups are referred to as *subcultures*. Subcultures are a part of a larger cultural group, but their distinctive ways of living make them a special subcultural group. Indeed, subcultures generally see themselves as part of the American culture, but they subscribe to some different values and ways of living which set them apart. For example, the hippies can be viewed as a subcultural group in our society with different norms of behavior. Nursing, too, is a subculture which has its own norms and practices that make it a special and distinct group. The subculture of nursing espouses norms which are somewhat different from those of other health professional groups such as social work and medicine. At the same time, the nursing subculture contains a number of norms which are part of the general American culture. Most assuredly, it is quite difficult for any subculture group to maintain its existence completely without reference to some of the cultural values and practices of the large culture to which they belong. This is especially true for professional groups since their services generally reflect the cultural norms of our large society—the American Culture.

American Cultural Values and Nursing

In this section, some of our major American cultural values will be highlighted and discussed in relation to their relevance to nursing. All too frequently, nurses, health workers, and other Americans are not fully aware of our own American cultural values and how these values influence their ways of thinking and acting. This is not too surprising since we (unconsciously) are so involved in living by our American values that we do not possess sufficient awareness and objectivity to know them in an explicit way. This is one reason why social scientists, more specifically anthropologists, specialize in the study and analysis of cultures and subculture groups.

Cultural values are a powerful force in governing man's behavior. Values have been defined as "directive elements which give order and direction to the ever-flowing stream of human acts and thoughts as they relate to the solution of common human problems."[12] The tenacity of cultural values, symbols, and action patterns cannot be underestimated, as one learns by coming to know and by working with people from different cultures. The values discussed below are some of the dominant American cultural values which influence our thinking and actions. Many of them are reflected in the subculture of nursing.

Cultural Value of Optimal Health. A cultural value of particular interest to health personnel is the heightened emphasis on *optimum health for all American citizens.* Good health is now a prescribed value and a right for people in our society. Ideally, no one is supposed to be denied optimal health; however, there are factors which limit the availability of health services to people. The maintenance of good health and the provision for a variety of health services for all Americans continues to be emphasized as a human right and a civil right for Americans by our federal, state, and local political and health-oriented leaders. Federal and state politicians are actively involved in emphasizing health program needs for all Americans. It is the talk and issue of our times.

Currently, the health emphasis is focused upon the aged, youth, and the "culturally disadvantaged and deprived" groups. The "culturally deprived" groups are seen largely as consisting of those who are economically and educationally deprived according to middle-class American norms. Many contend the "culturally deprived" have poor health practices. There are, however, some "culturally deprived" groups whose health practices are not as grave and deficient as they are assumed to be. Most important, the economically deprived cultural groups frequently have rich social and cultural ways of living by their kinship and religious practices. It is, therefore, unfortunate that so many cultural groups are being labeled "deprived" in a generalized way. The marked emphasis in our society upon the culture value of "optimum health" for all people is not only difficult and questionable to attain, it is a norm which is in sharp contrast with other cultures in the world. In some cultures, health is not one of the people's primary or major cultural values having an optimal health emphasis. Moreover, there may be limited financial, social, and political efforts expended by the people in these cultures for maintaining a high level of wellness. Instead, other cultural values such as environmental development may receive more attention than health. Within the United States, we have subculture groups who do not view health as their primary and major value, and so they are experiencing conflicts between their own particular subcultural values and those of the larger society. Thus the cultural value of optimum health in American society may vary in strength of belief and in realistic goal implementation. This point is extremely important for nurses and other health personnel to recognize in their often eager attempts to change the health practices of people in this country and abroad to their "optimal" perceived level.

In general, professional nurses and other health personnel tend to support the cultural value of optimum health, for it is viewed as their primary interest and their professional *raison d'etre*. Their desire for and eagerness to promote this professional health value among other cultural and subcultural groups whose health values differ significantly from theirs may well get in the way of being a helpful professional person. Certainly, it can be a major reason for inter- and intracultural group tensions and the reason why some cultural groups avoid health professionals or show limited interest in their health recommendations and practices. It is common practice for some cultural groups to show exterior signs of being polite, deferent, and passive toward professional health practitioners, but interiorly they may feel quite different. Different kinds of feelings such as anger and resentment may be found, and often the local people are afraid to express these feelings overtly to health personnel. This behavior becomes particularly evident when cultural groups quietly refuse to follow the health suggestions and practices of the professional group. In their non-verbal way, these cultural groups ponder over such questions as: What right do these professional people have to impose their health values on us? Don't they realize that we have our own cultural values regarding health? Why do they insist that we change our health values for theirs?

Most cultures and subcultures have their own health norms and practices —a fact often not realized or understood by health personnel. Consequently, indigenous groups wonder why they have to adopt new or different health-illness norms. They wonder why they must change their values to another set of values, especially if the new values are not congruent with their traditional beliefs and practices. It is no wonder that many cultural and subcultural groups in this country and abroad continue to use their own indigenous health practices after they have been exposed to or taught our professional health practices and values. Indeed, more knowledge and careful planning are needed in helping other cultures whose health emphases and values differ from ours. Some perceptive nurses, too, question their right to impose their health values and practices upon a cultural group who have a different health-illness system.

Cultural Value of Democracy. Our cultural heritage of being a democratic society pervades as an ideal norm of our culture. This ideal norm, however, may not be a manifest norm which is readily apparent to outsiders. A gap may exist between the believed-in and operational norms. Concepts, policies, and values inherent in the norm of democracy ideally emphasize social equality, equal representation in local, state, and federal governmental affairs, and equal rights for all Americans to participate in the American way of life. These democratic beliefs are supposed to operate in all of our educational, political, religious, and social institutions. The cultural ideal of democracy is often construed as meaning unrestrained freedom of speech and freedom of action in our society, and consequently responsibility for and sensitivity to the rights and needs of other cultural groups may not be fully recognized. Moreover, the cultural value of democracy may be in sharp contrast with people of other cultures or subcultural groups who live by norms associated with autocracy. It is important that health personnel recognize these cultural norm differences and identify ways to appropriately work with these cultures without undue imposition of one's own values upon another group.

The cultural norm of democracy is reflected in patient care and in educational practices in nursing. Numerous documentary examples could be given to show how democracy operates as both an ideal and manifest norm in nursing. For example, when nurses plan for and administer nursing care to patients, they often reveal a conviction that all patients in their unit should receive equal treatment and care, and that no patient is given more attention than another. Implicit with this behavior is the belief that it is not "democratic" or "fair" to treat patients differently, as all patients have the same democratic right to nursing care and the nurse has the obligation to fulfill this right. It is fascinating to observe how frequently nurses struggle to give an equal amount of time, care, and attention to all patients in "their district area", "their ward", or to "their assigned group." They express by their behavior that they are not favoring unduly one patient for another even though one patient may need considerably more time and attention than another patient because of his particular health problem or reaction to illness. Democratic norms are also seen operating in nursing education. Comments such as the following are frequently heard: "All nursing students should be given equal rights, equal participation, and equal consideration;" "A nurse is a nurse regardless of her professional experiences and educational preparation;" "We as nurses are all alike and equal;" "What is good for one nursing student or faculty member is democratically justified for another." Teachers in nursing often make great efforts to help each student in similar ways and try to give approximately the same amount of time and help to each student. They are careful not to show too much interest in any one student as they unconsciously anticipate repercussions related to student injustice and partiality as well as a feeling of violating democratic principles in educational practices. The author recalls faculty members stating this dictum which served as a guide to their teaching: "If you treat each student equally and in a similar way, you will never have trouble with your students."

The Cultural Value of Individualism. In the American culture, the rights and values of the individual are recognized and respected. Support of special interests, needs, and rights of individuals are not only expressed as an ideal norm to be fulfilled in our culture, but also have legal sanction. "Rugged individualism," an old cultural norm which continues to be upheld in our society, is exemplified by the individual who works very hard and achieves success. Considerable recognition and reward has been given to rugged individualism in our society. Recently, the concept and cultural value of individualism is receiving marked emphases regarding the particularistic and special rights of individuals from a legal, economic and social perspective. The individual is being perceived as a very special and unique human who can expect to receive individualized recognition and status in our culture. Marked emphasis upon individuals with their own personal rights, with their own property, and own legal and social rights can be noted (even with newborn infants) in our culture. Accordingly, one finds there is generally more attention given to the rights, welfare, and privileges of an individual than to that of a social group. People from other cultures who emphasize the importance of group values and rights are shocked to find the marked emphasis given to the individual in our culture. To some of these strangers it appears to be a marked narcissistic focus. The culture value of individualism is buttressed in our society by our religious beliefs and practices, political decisions, individualized economic pursuits, and personalized social interests. For example in our religious practices as found in Roman Catholic teachings, the unique rights, dignity, and freedom of the individual as a human being are emphasized. Infants, adolescents, and adults as individuals in our culture must be recognized and legally protected. Today, laws are being established in many states to protect the individual rights of infants and small children from adult abuse. In contrast, some cultures do not have laws to protect each child, nor do some cultures even contemplate the need for such a law as their attitude toward children differs considerably from ours, and is focused upon needs of groups in their society.

The cultural ideal of marked individualism appears at times to be in direct conflict with the ideal of democracy, which stresses equal rights to all. How can an individual's rights be fully expressed and recognized when democratic principles stress the social equality and the equal rights of *all* people in our society? Americans continue to deal with these two value conflicts so that both values are sustained and lived by. To deal with this problem, Americans have learned a variety of ways to interpret, explain, or rationalize their actions and intellectual discourses regarding individualism and democracy, so that the values are preserved. Sometimes Americans deal with these values by ranking them according to a first or second priority and according to the situation and the way the situation can be logically and empirically defended.

This American focus upon the individual and his rights, freedom, and personal welfare, is in sharp contrast with many cultures of the world which tend to give tacit recognition to the individual but substantive recognition to social groups. In many non-Western societies, the social group always has a higher status and more rights than any individual. In these societies, the individual is in a subordinate position and receives less respect and consideration than the social group.

The cultural value of giving emphasis to the person as an individual being is certainly found in nursing. The ideal norm in nursing has long been to provide highly individualized and personalized care to patients. Each patient treated in the hospital, clinic, or community agency is generally given full consideration as an individual in staff conferences and in the nurse's efforts to provide individualized nursing care. Only very recently have group nursing plans and group care been given study and consideration, and this has occurred mainly in psychiatric nursing. Seldom does one find the practice of nurses focusing primarily upon the needs or problems of a group of patients. Invariably, nurses tend to consider each individual patient—his own rights, needs and welfare. Even in community health nursing, where the nurse is expected to focus upon the total family and community as a functioning social unit, there is a tendency for the nurse to focus upon one member of the family and this individual's needs and problems become highlighted with only a cursory treatment of family group dynamics and health practices. The family's health needs and planning tends to be done with respect to one patient's needs and goals. Thus, the practice of nursing today remains largely focused upon the health needs and problems of individual patients. With the current trend toward community and ecological health problems, it will be of interest to see if there will be a shift in the nursing care cultural norms from the individual to the large community group. Historically, the American Nurses' Association has stressed in its code of nursing practice the importance of recognizing individual rights and needs of patients. Recently, this Association has issued a statement to further protect the human rights and welfare of individual patients or clients subjected to research study.

The Cultural Value of Achieving and Doing. Achieving and doing are interrelating cultural values which are highly emphasized in our culture, and especially by middle-class Americans. Generally, successful people are viewed as those individuals who work hard, keep busy, and try hard to reach the top. Success is a goal which many Americans believe can only be achieved by action and constant awareness of ways to achieve this goal. EACH YEAR Americans feel they should be increasing their salary earnings, improving their job situation, and moving forward on the social, political and economic ladder. The cultural value of achievement keeps a person moving or doing something to convince others of his respectable motives and sincere worth. The desire for personal advancement and success appear to be the underlying drive for achieving and doing. Achievement usually involves competition and high expectations of oneself and others. This cultural value has its consequences, too, in that many middle class Americans appear to be under considerable pressure to achieve or do something and to find relaxation difficult. Americans appear to be resorting more and more to medicinal aids, drugs, and alcohol to help them relax and to alleviate daily stresses and problems. Somatic illness manifestations are often associated with the consequences of stress, high achievement expectations and keeping extremely involved in doing something.

The cultural value of achieving and doing is noticeably manifest in nursing. Traditionally, our professional efforts and goals have largely been action-oriented. The predominant image held by nurses and the public is that the nurse is a "doer," a professional person who is constantly in action or ready to take action in helping patients with their physical or psychological needs. In both education and practice much emphasis has been given to the nurse achieving certain specified goals and accomplishing specified tasks related to patient care. Many nurses feel they are not being "good nurses" unless they are doing something concrete for others or keeping physically active. For the nurse, to be primarily in an active listening or thinking role as a primary and important part of nursing practice is still difficult for many nurses to accept because action appears to be the chief *modus operandus* and role behavior of a nurse. There is, however, in this "modern" era of nursing, much being said about the professional nurse becoming more a thinker, planner, and assessor of health care than a physically action-oriented person who must keep physically busy. Social, economic, political, and professional forces in nursing are shaping the nursing profession so that the achievement (and doing) cultural value will be brought in line with the value of thinking and critical intellectualism. There is also an encouraging trend today, in raising the professional status of nursing through knowledgeable nursing actions and understanding sociocultural forces influencing nursing directions.

The Cultural Value of Cleanliness. For middle and middle-upper class Americans, cleanliness is next to godliness. Cleanliness is a dominant culture value, which is closely related to the values of optimum health and physical aesthetics. Much of our time is lavished upon washing our hands, taking baths, washing clothes, scrubbing and keeping the house clean, disposing of trash, and so on. Children are reprimanded if they are dirty, and often they receive rather severe punishment when found soiled. Many of the advertisements on television and the radio are directed toward urging us to keep ourselves, our neighborhoods, and our country clean, neat, and tidy. Moreover, millions of dollars are spent each year on keeping America clean, keeping trash in proper receptacles, and keeping our public rest rooms and eating facilities clean. In fact, keeping America clean has received recent emphasis and was one of the chief interest of the wife of a former President of the United States, Mrs. Lyndon B. Johnson. A beautiful, clean, and tidy American country is an ideal norm of our society. Few countries in the world are so concerned about national cleanliness and keeping our homes immaculately clean and the country sides tidy as Americans. In fact, visitors from foreign cultures are often amazed to find so much stress upon cleanliness and how many Americans seem to order their lives aroudn the value of keeping physically clean and tidy. With some cultural groups, the people contend there are positive health values in direct exposure to dirt and in remaining a bit unclean. Such conflicts in cultural values may be difficult for health personnel to understand and to adjust to as they work with people who do not maintain high standards of cleanliness.

The value of cleanliness is highly evident in nursing. Nurses spend considerable time keeping the patient clean and keeping the patient's immediate physical environment tidy and clean. Keeping patients clean is viewed as enhancing the optimum health state of the patient. The germ-free concept which began during the asepsis era in medicine has been retained by health personnel as an important principle of and ideal for good health. It is believed that if the patient and his environment are kept physically clean, the patient will have a good probability of remaining healthy and well. Accordingly, the nurse and her assistants are the key health persons to keep the patient clean and they are usually rewarded by positive comments and rewards from their superiors if they maintain cleanliness and are attentive to the asepsis principle in giving patient care. Sometimes physical cleanliness supersedes the importance of the interpersonal, cultural, and social needs of patients. The recent trend in nursing aims to help nurses realize that interpersonal, social, and psychological care of patients is equally as important as keeping the patient physically clean and neat.

The Cultural Value of Time. The American culture gives much emphasis to the concept and use of time. Time is a dominant value to Americans, so much so that their lives are largely regulated and dictated by the clock. Time has economic, political, and social values, and so it is extremely important to us. To many middle-class Americans, time must not be wasted, but always used well and effectively. Time dictates where one should be each hour of the day, and sometimes at night. Typically, the middle-class American often feels guilty and regretful if he is not busy and maintaining his time schedule. Time can even cause serious accidents and contribute to physical, social, and mental illnesses. Thus time largely regulates the course of our lives and strongly influences our well-being. It is precious and difficult to use judiciously in our society.

In many cultures of the world, time does not have such importance in people's lives, and so people are not slaves to clocks and time schedules. Some cultures do not even possess a time instrument or know what one is like. For example, the Gadsup people of New Guinea had never seen a clock or watch until the anthropologist showed them one. However, they do gain some general indication of how time is lapsing from the position of the sun and activities completed during a day. Since time does not dominate the Gadsup way of life, one finds their mental, physical, and cultural health status quite different from Americans, and mainly because they are not under the constant pressure of routinizing their lives by a time instrument.

There are a number of ways that the cultural value of time regulates the nurse's life and care of patients. Most obvious, are the precise times in which medicines and treatment procedures should be administered by the nurse. Physicians' visits, nursing care conferences, patients' meals, shift reports, home visits, and many other activities have a time assigned to them and regulate the nurse's activities in a hospital setting. They determine where the nurse should be at certain times of the day or evening and what she should be doing at certain time intervals. Time determines how much care and attention she can offer each patient, the physician, and other health workers. With the current emphases upon precise time that medications and treatments can be given to affect optimal therapeutic results, the nurse is becoming increasingly sensitive to the concept of time and its assumed importance in affecting the health status of a patient. Time does largely govern the nurse's activities and functions with patients and also greatly determines her educational goals and professional career opportunities. The nurse is highly sensitive to time cues and the consequences of time upon the health status of people.

The Cultural Value of Automation. During the past decade, the cultural norm of technology and the concomitant impact of automation have become markedly evident in our American way of life. Automation has drastically changed our patterns of living. It has influenced health practices, modified social relationships, and changed occupational and social roles of men, women, and children. Automation has created an employment shortage for three million unskilled Americans, and yet a crisis exists in the lack of highly skilled manpower to develop new machines and maintain existing ones.[13] As we know, many tasks which were once performed by unskilled and semi-skilled workers are now performed by automatic electric and nuclear machines. Our attitudes and expectations about machine efficiency and productivity can be readily noted. At the same time, we are aware of some of the emerging positive and negative consequences of the machine. For example, man's growing tendency to relate to machines more than gaining satisfaction from human interactions. Americans expect machines to perform instantly and effectively and if this does not occur, we are quickly annoyed and impatient with machines. Furthermore, only the latest and best equipment is desired by most middle and upper-class Americans. The latest machine on the market is believed to be the "best" and is actively sought for by the machine-oriented man or woman. This behavioral expectation is expressed in a familiar statement: "We must keep up to date by having the latest and the best technological items in our hospitals, homes, business places, and institutions." American advertising agencies support the use of automatic or technical machines and devices through our mass communication media. As interactional processes change from person-to-person contacts to person-to-machine, one finds signs of depersonalization in human relationships occurring, and especially in health care practices. However, the ideal norm in nursing is still to preserve personalized modes of interaction with patiens as much as possible.

How is modern technology influencing man's future and his survival? From an anthropological perspective, man can and does determine the development of technology and he can control the use of technologies. Concommitantly, man must give thought to how our technological way of life may helpfully serve man in a constructive way or lead to the destruction of man in a precipitious or unintentional manner. We know that by merely pressing an atomic button, it is possible to annihilate the human species as well as all subhuman species. The problem of life and/or the extinction of the human race depends largely on man's decisions, behavior and wisdom. The evolution of man has been in process for millions of years; however, man's technological inventions have increased rapidly and impressively and are almost beyond his full comprehension and complete control. Is it time to give serious thought and planning to the direction and constructive use of modern technology for the future? The consequences of technological automation affects not only our American society but also other cultures of the world. Thus the cross-cultural ethical aspects of what technologies should or should not be developed and their constructive uses is a topic of interest to all men in the world.

Although many statements could be made about the ways modern technology is shaping nursing, only a few will be cited as there is a growing body of available literature regarding this subject.[14][15] A variety of computers are being used in hospitals and public health agencies to quickly collate health data and services in patient care and treatment. It is predicted that most hospital and other kinds of health institutions will have computers for practically everything. Automatic treatment machines for the treatment of heart, lung, and kidney conditions are already in use and more efficient machines are being produced. Such automatic devices and many others are rapidly becoming a part of the nurse's environment today. How is the role of the nurse changing with automation? What will be the nurse's role for the future in a technologically advanced society? What changes will there be in the patient's expectations of the nurse because of automation? These and other questions are currently being studied by nurses and her technology colleagues.

It is the author's belief that no matter how efficient and effective machines may be in health treatment, there will still remain an extremely important area of responsibility for the nurse to meet the predicted increased need of people for humanistic and personalized individual and group care in our society. If the nurse is content to permit or assume that the machine will take over this aspect of care, she (he) is missing an important understanding about man's fundamental human needs and tendencies. If a perceptive nurse carefully observes people receiving "machine care", she will note the areas which more than ever need the nurse's professional skills in interpersonal relationships related to reduction of anxiety, stress, and fear of complex machines. In contrast to Bennett's position in a recent article, this author contends that nursing will not become extinct with modern technologies in the future unless the nurse permits herself to become insensitive to man's human and interpersonal psychosocial and cultural needs.[16] Bennett's article fails to recognize the many sociocultural and emotional needs of patients exposed to machines. There are no machines today which come near to fulfilling these critical and important needs of man. It is, indeed, the challenge of nursing practices during this heightened use of technology in patient care to recognize the psychological, social and cultural support of patients. In sum, this chapter has exposed the reader to a beginning exploration of American cultural values in order to help nurses understand how our cultural values influence health trends and nursing practices. Cultural values are not only guidelines for health practice, but are crucial to understanding people and health behavior.

FOOTNOTES

[1] Another version of this chapter was given as the keynote address for the Annual Work Conference of the Minnesota League for Nursing, February 1, 1968, where it was entitled "The Significance of Cultural Concepts in Nursing." Reported in the Minnesota League for Nursing Bulletin, July 1968, Vol. XVI, No. 3, 3-12.

[2] Margaret Mead, *Sex and Temperament in Three Primitive Societies*, New York, 1935, p. 322.

[3] Benjamin Paul, *Health, Culture and Community*, New York: Russell Sage Foundation, 1955.

[4] *Ibid.*

[5] Edward H. Spicer (Ed.), *Human Problems in Technological Change*, New York: Russell Sage Foundation, 1952.

[6]Saunders, Lyle, *Cultural Differences and Medical Care*, New York: Russell Sage Foundation, 1954.
[7]Madeleine Leininger, "Study of Social Science Courses Taught in Baccalaureate and Graduate NLN Accredited Schools of Nursing in the United States," unpublished research report, 1968.
[8]A. L. Kroeber and Clyde Kluckhohn, *Culture: A Critical Review of Concepts and Definitions*, PPMAAW, XLVII, No. 1, Cambridge, 1952.
[9]Melville J. Herskovits, *Cultural Anthropology*, New York: Alfred A. Knopf, 1955, p. 305.
[10]*Ibid*, p. 306.
[11]Leslie A. White, *The Evolution of Culture*, New York: McGraw-Hill Book Company, Inc., 1958, p. 8.
[12]Florence Kluckhohn, *Variations in Value Orientations*, Evanston, Illinois, 1961, p. 4.
[13]John Tebbel, "People and Jobs," *Saturday Review*, December, 1967, p. 8.
[14]Betty Jane Tarrant, "Automation, Its Effect on the Patient, *American Journal of Nursing*, October, 1966, pp. 2190-2194.
[15]Robert L. Rowen, "Automation, Its Effect on the Hospital," *American Journal of Nursing*, October 1966, p. 2199.
[16]Leland R. Bennett, "This I Believe ... That Nurses May Become Extinct," *Nursing Outlook*, January, 1970, Vol. 18 p. 28-32.

5 The Traditional Culture of Nursing and the Emerging New One

It is a point worthy of reflection that to date there has been no anthropological description or formulation of the subculture of nursing, and yet a culture of nursing does exist now, as it has in the past.[1] The traditional culture of nursing is changing and a new emerging culture can be identified. But before discussing these two cultures of nursing, we will explore some of the reasons why the culture of nursing has not been identified or studied until the present time.

The first and most obvious reason why there has been no description of or formulation about the culture of nursing is the paucity of nurse-anthropologists in the field and those interested in this topic. It is true that there have been a few non-nurse anthropologists involved in nursing, but their interest has not been sufficiently strong to study this aspect of nursing. Secondly, even if some anthropologists would have been interested in studying the culture of nursing, they might have been reluctant to pursue the task. In presenting the culture of nursing both the favorable and the unfavorable features of nursing would need to be reported, and there might have been a reluctance by anthropologists to give such a report of a professional group. It is, nevertheless, important to reveal "things as they are" and not to disguise facts because a group may be uncomfortable with them. Both the overt and covert aspects of the nursing profession must be examined in order to provide an objective and accurate picture of the nursing culture. A nurse-anthropologist who is keenly aware of the profession and who maintains a high degree of objectivity in her study of the nursing culture can offer rich insights into the profession. It would, however, be interesting to have a non-nurse anthropologist examine the nursing culture, and to check these findings with those of a nurse-anthropologist.

As the author investigated the subculture of nursing, the participant-observational field study method was used as well as structured and open informal interviews with a variety of key informants in nursing across the United States. Both the longitudinal and horizontal perspectives of nursing contributed to the formulation of the cultures of nursing. In addition, the author's twenty-three years of experience in the field of nursing in different kinds of nursing institutions and in different geographical settings provided first-hand data about generalized and specific features of nursing to make empirical and inferred statements about the old and the new cultures of nursing.

Formulations about the culture of nursing can be viewed as primarily major themes of nursing behavior, that is, the recurrent and standardized patterns of behavior shown by nurses at different general periods of time in nursing. The intent was to provide a generalized profile of the cultures of nursing so that interested persons could obtain an overall view of the major cultural patterns or themes of nursing. It should help nurses to understand their own subculture of nursing and may provide a comparative picture of nursing with other groups. Nurses have been interested in their own professional image to recruit people into the field and to influence relationships with other professional and non-professional groups. Formulations about the cultural norms and values of a profession may help newcomers into the nursing profession as well as those already in the field to understand the major characteristics of the nursing profession.

A description of the culture of nursing makes one realize that the nursing profession socializes its members to meet certain implicit and explicit normative expectations. Actually, a sizeable volume could be written about the culture of nursing, but for the purposes of this book, only a few cardinal featues have been presented. Many of the highly idiosyncratic or particularistic aspects of nurse behavior have not been included. This does not mean that these aspects are not important as frequently idiosyncratic behavior becomes clues to changes in the norms of a professional group, or they may represent major conflicts among and between norms. Interestingly enough, the author found far more general and uniform features of nursing behavior through her study than highly idiosyncratic or divergent behavioral tendencies. There are, however, more noticeable signs of divergent tendencies emerging since 1965.

In the process of analyzing the culture of nursing, the data fell into two broad ethnological divisions, namely, the traditional culture of nursing and the emerging new culture of nursing. These two contrasting categories were derived from the cognitive statements and behavior of nurses as they spoke about these "old and new ways of nursing." Thus these categories and some of the raw statements of behavior regarding each category were used by nurses as they talked about themselves and the nursing profession. The author then synthesized and made refined formulations about clusters of these behavioral descriptions.

One of the crucial aspects influencing the conceptualization of the two cultures was the perception of the culture of nursing derived from the hospital educational preparation (the old culture) and that of nursing derived from learning in institutions of higher education (the new culture). The dichotomization of perceptions and conceptualizations along these two lines was fairly unequivocal and descriptive of each culture.

Before presenting the culture of nursing, a few preface comments are in order to orient the reader to the cultural formulations. First, there may be a tendency for the reader to "read-in" or infer ethical and moral judgments about the statements, or to assign a "right" or "wrong" value judgment to the ethnographic statements. It is important to state that the ethnographer was not interested in judging whether the behavior modalities of the old or new culture of nursing are right or wrong. Rather, the intent is to describe and explain the existing formulations about the culture of nursing. The author must present the behavior of nurses as it was made evident by the methods used in the study. Secondly, as the reader studies the traditional and emerging cultures of nursing it is advisable not to rigidly categorize all nurses as belonging to one culture or the other. Most nurses have attributes of both cultures; it is, however, conceivable that some nurses' behavior does veer toward one culture more than the other. Moreover, some nurses may verbally espouse the beliefs of the emerging culture, yet manifest behavior of the traditional culture. Moreover, the chronological age of the nurse does not determine if the nurse "belongs" to the traditional or emerging culture. It is the manifest or total constellation of behavior of the nurse that is important in determining her identification with these two cultures of nursing. And, lastly, the author does not want to imply that one culture is better or worse than the other. Such a judgment may vary with each nurse's philosophical beliefs as well as with each professional subgroup of nurses.

Other-Directed and Self-Directed Behaviors

One of the outstanding features of the traditional culture of nursing was the tendency of nurses to be *other-directed*. Reisman's concept of the "other directed" person helps to describe the behavior of traditional nurses, whose behavior revealed that they were inclined to be guided largely by the beliefs, actions, and norms of an outside reference group.[2] Only quite recently are nurses beginning to assert behavior which reveals autonomy in thinking and practice and behavior, that differs from patterns of thinking found in the medical profession. Nurses are becoming less disposed to follow the practice patterns of physicians and more inclined to develop their own beliefs about nursing and ways to become an autonomous and distinct profession. An examination of nursing textbooks and periodicals from 1925 to 1950 shows clearly the strong influence of the medical profession upon nursing education and practice. There remain, however, several schools of nursing that follow the old culture of nursing and continue to pattern their clinical experiences and educational programs upon the norms of the field of medicine. With the new culture, one finds nurses challenging the beliefs and practices of the medical profession as to their relevance to nursing practice, and they are testing new models for professional nursing education and practice. Certainly in the past, nursing was influenced not only by the medical profession but also by the expectations and demands of hospital administrators. The nursing profession as a predominantly female profession has experienced the control and power of male professional and occupational groups, such as medicine and hospital administration. Consequently, some female nursing groups were treated as subordinate persons to males and were subject to their thinking and demands. Presently, one of the primary problems of the nursing profession is to address itself to equal recognition and rights for female professional women in the labor field and to examine discriminatory practices which limit nurses from achieving recognition and top positions in the health field. It is quite evident that the nursing profession was under the power, control, and dominance of the medical profession. Now nurses are turning to deal with problems related to shared power, shared authority, and shared decision-making, with members of the medical profession in order to optimize their contribution to patient care. This is another sign of the new culture of nursing as it moves from being less other-directed to that of being more self-directed.

In the process of becoming more self-directed and more autonomous in thinking and actions than in the past, one can note through the literature and in conferences that nurses desire to formulate their own body of knowledge about nursing.[3] Most important, nurses are actively trying to develop this body of knowledge through clinical research studies and critical study of specific nursing interventions. With the new culture of nursing, nursing is trying to change its norms of practice, its traditional image, and its modes of practice with other professional groups. The growing number of nurses prepared through master and doctoral programs are providing leadership for the new culture. It is viewed as a timely movement in light of current challenges in the nursing profession and the national health challenge for better health care and delivery of health services to people. Thus the gradual shift from the traditional subcultural norm of being largely other-directed and by the norms of the medical profession to that of becoming more self-directed appears to characterize the evolving new culture of nursing.

Paternalism, Self-Sacrifice, and Self-Needs

Traditionally, the culture of nursing was marked by the qualities of *paternalism, self-sacrifice, and self-dedication.* Paternalism was revealed in the way nurses showed deference to father-like protective figues, such as a physician. The value placed on protection, guidance, and accepting "fatherly" suggestions from men was evidence in the early traditions of nursing. Nurses seemed to bask in the paternalism provided by persons in superordinate positions or those who had a paternalistic attitude toward the nurse. Frequently, physicians, hospital administrators, and the directors of special health programs were persons who took a warm paternalistic and protective interest in nurses. Accordingly, the reciprocal behavior of the nurse toward these paternal figures was one of submission, deference, respect, and acceptance. Traditionally, nurses have been socialized to be quiet and humble in the presence of father-like authority figures and their behavior revealed signs of respect, attention, and reverence to them. There has also been a past tendency for nurses to confide in those individuals who were paternalistic, and then to reciprocally offer these persons special favors, considerations, and maternal-like care. If the nurse did not show deferent behavior to paternalistic figures, she could not expect to be helped in crisis situations nor to receive protection in emergency situations that involved her. Dependence upon persons in authority and deference to those with paternalistic interests in nurses was an early distinct characteristic of the traditional culture of nursing.

Today, in the emerging culture of nursing, paternalism is waning and nurses are becoming more independent and self-sufficient. As a consequence, they are relying upon their own professional group for self-development, growth, and protection of their rights. Lately, one can detect symptoms of some physicians experiencing "cultural shock" as the nurse does not respond to the physicians' requests in a totally accepting and deferent manner. The nurse is exhibiting independent thinking and decision-making as she cares for patients. To some physicians, this behavior is shocking and reveals a drastic shift from the time when nurse functioned assiduously as the "handmaid" and "perpetual servant" to the physician. Overt hostility and attempts to control nursing educational programs and clinical practice have been part of the recent response of some physicians to counteract the nurses' independent thinking and action. Thus the shift in the nurse's behavior to become independent and self-guided has been a noticeable change for colleagues who have traditionally perceived the nurse as a dependent figure highly responsive to paternalism.

In examining numerous examples of the traditional nurse-physician relationships, one realizes how much nurses have always been direct assistants to physicians and have been guided by their thinking and needs. As several nurses of the old culture stated, "We met all their requests. We not only took care of their patients, but also cared for them. We seldom questioned the physicians' directions and need for care." Examples of "caring for" the physician were: stacking the physician's charts, writing special notes (in addition to the nursing care notes) for the physician, providing a special and quiet place for him to work when he came on the ward, offering him coffee or breakfast, obtaining special instruments for the physician to examine "his" patients, and making rounds with him to see "his" patients. These caring tasks provided by nurses for physicians were ritualized and sanctioned in most institutions and did take considerable professional nursing time—time which today is being gradually used for patient care. Today, in private hospitals, one can find evidence of the nurse still providing caring tasks for the physician, the hospital administrator, and the patient. In these settings, the care of the physician continues to take much of the nurse's time and efforts; however, nurses of the new culture are quite aware of this past expected norm of behavior and are trying to change this practice.

Closely related to paternalism in nursing were the traditional cultural values of *self-sacrifice and self-dedication to others.* In its early history, nursing was viewed primarily as a vocation and a calling, and so the nurse was expected to be a public and self-dedicated servant. Nursing was viewed largely as a religious calling dedicated to help God through others, and so the nurse gave of herself untiringly, and sacrificed many personal needs for humanitarian and Christian service. Accordingly, many nursing practices and norms evolved from religious ideas and from deplorable social conditions and necessities. The phrase "the nurse is an angel of mercy" reflected the spiritual, mystical, and self-dedicated service of the nurse to the sick and needy. The cultural norm in the traditional culture of nursing included not only dedication and self-sacrifice, but also virtue. A highly virtuous woman was perceived as being altruistic, self-dedicated, and maintaining a sense of "purity." The Nightingale pledge which stated, "I solemnly pledge myself before God and in the presence of this assembly to pass my life in purity and to practice my profession faithfully ..," embodied some of the virtuous expectations of the nurse. Indeed, the "Florence Nightingale nurse" of the past was expected to be self-sacrificing to both God and man by remaining morally fit, pure, faithful, reliable, and a "good nurse." Miss Nightingale stressed in her writings and practice the qualities of sympathy, gentleness, devotion to others, and loyalty as the important qualities for nurses. In the traditional culture, the nurse was expected to work long hours (often 12-18 hours per day) for this was symbolically a sign of her dedication to others and ability to withstand work expectations for the "common good" of the profession. The implicit cultural norm was that the nurse would seldom complain about onerous situations or difficult tasks, because she was expected to tolerate self-discomfort and stress while helping others. This completely self-sacrificing attitude of the nurse sounds akin to masochistic behavior, in which an individual tends to accept heavy demands and punishment from another person. The nurse of the traditional nursing culture was capable of giving to others without revealing her own personal needs, problems, or discomforts. Moreover, she could manage to give good nursing care with very limited equipment and often poor facilities, and she was amazingly adept at improvising procedures and adjusting to situations with minimal complaints. How frequently nurses of the old culture said they had to use second-hand materials and then creatively devised new equipment and new techniques in order to provide care to patients. One can see the positive values in these norms which required that the nurse be a highly innovative person, able to adjust to many difficult situations.

With the new culture of nursing, the philosophy, spirit, and practice of nursing is changing. Today, the nurse perceives herself as a professional person who provides health services to others in relation to her professional preparation, needs, and life situation. Of most importance, *the nurse's needs, interests, and goals are receiving much recognition and consideration as an essential part of becoming a* successful nurse. Nursing as a "vocational calling" is rapidly changing to the idea that nursing is a highly professional field with business and occupational interests. Nurses are negotiating for satisfactory working conditions, a livable salary, and labor rights and benefits equal to other occupational or labor groups. The nurse today expects modern equipment and supplies to give care to patients, and not to be handicapped by inadequate equipment. The provision of comfort measures for nurses in the hospitals or health agencies is now a necessary requirement to retain nurses. The number of nursing staff and their preparation are also being assessed by nurses as they seek a new position so that they can be reasonably assured of giving adequate care to patients and will not be frustrated by a low patient-staff ratio. Fringe and regular employment benefits are expected by the qualified professional nurse if the employer wishes to retain her. In general, there has been a noticeable shift in the value orientation of professional nurses from that of being almost completely self-sacrificing and dedicated to others to that of being concerned about one's own welfare and only reasonably or limitedly dedicated to others. Indeed, the nurse's *own* interests are receiving much attention because it is believed that if her own needs and interests are not reasonably met, the nurse will not be an effective person with patients. Consequently, with the recent focus upon the nurse's needs, the nurse is becoming more articulate about her problems and concerns as she cares for patients and works with other staff members in an institution. There are also many opportunities for the nurse to communicate her needs and problems to others through formal or informal means in most health agencies. Active collective bargaining by nurses, protest marching, and special requests for modern economic security programs for nurses also reflect a definite change toward norms of an emerging new culture of nursing. The individual nurse as well as the total professional nursing group are being considered in the economic security programs for nurses. Demands for adequate salaries, shorter work hours, optimal working conditions, and economic security benefits are some of the recent norm expectations of the nurse today and contrast sharply with the Christian and self-sacrificing norms of the past.

The "successful nurse" in the new culture is being recognized as the nurse who can articulate and knowledgeably communicate her problems and needs to others so that effective care to patients can be given. This nurse is also expected to be a change agent to modify patterns of patient care in health care nursing systems. In all this change, there are nevertheless nurses who espouse to the values of the traditional culture and seriously question the current changes in nursing values. To these nurses, the new cultural norms are not only questionable but are affecting the "true essence and character of professional nursing."

Authoritarian and Democratic Values

Nurses of the traditional culture are keenly aware of the cultural norm of authoritarianism and the current emphases for democratic practices in health settings and schools of nursing. They speak of positive and negative features of authoritarianism as it prevailed in the past. Authoritarianism principles in the past provided protection and unquestionable guidelines regarding sources of authority and compliance of one's behavior toward persons in authority. Many of these nurses contend that controlled guidance and knowledge of who is in authority gave them a sense of personal security, protection, and established directions of communication. At the same time, nurses of the traditional culture recognized that strong authoritarian behavior generally suppressed freedom of thinking and the opportunity to act upon one's own hunches or beliefs. As a consequence, nurses were inclined to be passive and compliant to their superiors and learned to accept situations as they were in the hospitals or schools. Nurses of the past are quick, however, to comment that the perceived weak authority of today produces a sense of insecurity in nurses and confusion rather than a sense of direction. They find that the vagueness of a "soft" democratic leader creates problems and perpetuates ambiguities regarding professional directions.

In the traditional culture, nursing leaders in education and service who espoused to authoritarian beliefs and action patterns expected nurses in subordinate roles to show respect and deference to others. Seldom did the nurse question an authoritarian leader, since her decisions and statements were viewed as a precedent which one was expected to follow. While nurses held these leaders in awe and respected them, nurses also feared these leaders mainly because of their power and control over them by virtue of their position. Nurses did not usually maintain a social relationship with an authoritarian leader, because an "equal interaction role" on a social basis seemed incompatible with their other leader-follower role expectations of one another. Authoritarian nurses and physician leaders were generally viewed as possessing complete and absolute knowledge of the health field, and seldom were they considered capable of making errors in their work. The power of persons in authority roles was often distorted much beyond that which a leader may ever have expected, desired, or anticipated; however, there seemed to be a need to perceive authority figures as strong and powerful leaders. Nurses were afraid to question or disagree with authority figures in the past and if a nurse did question them, she did so with extreme caution and humbleness.

The traditional attitudes of nurses toward persons in authority were easy to observe in school and hospital situations. Physicians, nursing service directors, nursing educators, and hospital administrators in authority roles were always recognized by letting them enter a room before the staff nurse or instructor. These leaders were expected to step into an elevator, or to enter the patient's room before anyone else in a subordinate role to them. Seldom did one speak before a person in such an authority role had spoken. In dining places, persons in authority and those who had status in the institution had their own special dining area, and tables which were marked to recognize their role and position in the system. In general, nurses of the traditional culture learned to be deferent and obedient to those in authority. They highly respected persons in an authority role and seemed to fear situations which might be figuratively "stepping on their superior's toes.' Many nurses were unable to deal directly with and talk openly about authority problems. They did, however, try to cope with such problems in a careful and humble manner.

The new emerging culture of nursing reveals a noticeable change in the picture just portrayed, especially wth regard to authority and democratic decision-making. Democratic principles are becoming more a part of nursing service and education, and highly authoritarian behavior is being questioned and revoked by young nurses. There are, however, obvious signs of tension and unresolved problems in institutional settings which reveal conflicts between the old and the new concepts of authority and democracy. Consequently, the young graduate of the nursing program may often be frustrated, angry, and restless with centers retaining authoritarian norms. It is, indeed, fascinating to observe how young nursing students and staff nurses spontaneously voice their views about a problem or topic under discussion to those in superordinate positions. Nurses today challenge many ideas, question past beliefs, and strive to have their ideas fully recognized. More and more, nurses are becoming less hesitant in approaching superiors or any persons in authority positions. Nurses of the new culture support democratic principles and insist that decisions are made by the group and not by the one or two persons in superior positions. They also expect frequent "feedback" about their ideas from their associates and leaders. Nurses of this culture expect that their leaders will be approachable and comfortable in social situations whether at work or at home. They are quite eager to discover their own abilities and work on their self-development with progressive and "open-minded intellectual leaders" in the field.

In schools of nursing (which are rapidly being located within institutions of higher education) one finds collegiate-oriented students most vocal in discussing their ideas about authoritarian and democratic behavior systems. Nursing students of the new culture have ideas about the kind of leadership which will permit them to function well and they are sensitive to institutional settings that thwart their full professional development. Naturally, there are nurses in some of our service and educational settings who are not comfortable with the democratic ideas of recent graduates of nursing programs, and so problems and conflicts are evident. The author has noted the trend for these new graduates to accept positions in new community health settings, as there is more freedom to function in a democratic way than in some hospital settings. But looking at the overall picture and trends, the democratic philosophy of education, service, and patient care appears to be gaining allegiance. The development of the individual and the opportunity for nurses to participate in their own life decisions and to form their own goals is becoming more the accepted cultural norm in professional work than the authoritarian norms of the past.

Doing versus Intellectual Norms

In the traditional culture, nursing was largely learned by the apprenticeship method which required that the novice in nursing observe and follow the behavior of her knowledgeable superiors. The nurse was taught the techniques and art of nursing by experienced nurses, physicians, and other personnel in the hospital setting. The "good" nurse in the traditional culture was one who could give direct care to patients by applying the techniques and skills she learned from experienced nurses. The nurse was inclined to do many physical comfort activities for a patient and to take care of his immediate situational needs. "Learning by doing" was the principle and desired method of learning "good" nursing care. In the traditional culture of nursing there was limited emphasis upon highly intellectual interests or upon the discovery of new nursing knowledge by critical thinking, reading, and experimental research studies. The study of clinical problems in depth and from a nursing research focus was not encouraged. Nurses were generally expected to follow prescribed patterns of nursing care and the "doctor's orders." There was limited emphases upon raising critical questions about nursing practices or to discover new patterns of care. Efficiency in the practice and standardization of techniques in nursing were the predominant norms in the traditional culture of nursing, except for some of the early innovative practices by Florence Nightingale and other early practitioners who contributed to the "early modern era" of nursing.[4]

With the emerging new culture of nursing which has been evolving since 1955, emphasis is being placed upon the creative "thinker" of nursing practice and less emphasis is given to being the continuous "doer." Nurses are being prepared to read extensively, to think critically about new approaches to nursing problems, to question practices, and to use problem-solving skills in arriving at new solutions to all problems. Independent thinking and creative leadership to solve nursing problems are being emphasized in the new culture of nursing.

The rapid explosion of knowledge in the health sciences has stimulated the professional nurse to gain as much knowledge as possible about a topic under study. In addition, research approaches and methods of studying health problems are encouraging the nurse to be an active researcher in the health field. Both undergraduate and graduate nurses are taught research methods; consequently, nurses are becoming active participants in the pursuit of new nursing knowledge and in testing ideas about nursing. They are also being encouraged to use multiple human resources to study nursing problems. The existence of multiple and complex factors influencing the health state of a patient is being realized more in the new nursing culture.

With these developments, collegiate nurses are being encouraged to become researchers, independent thinkers, and reactors to different theories and practices. Nursing educators are helping students to construct and test theoretical ideas in relation to nursing practice. In general, there is considerable freedom and opportunity to examine the nurse's hunches and ideas about improving patient care.

Even though these behavioral modalities are becoming part of the emerging culture of nursing, there are still a number of schools and hospital systems which look askance at these emerging norms. People in some nursing settings are dubious as to whether the nurse of tomorrow will be able to give adequate care if she is more of a thinker than a doer. They contend that the recent graduate of collegiate nursing programs has limited technical skills and practical knowledge in caring for the patient's physical needs. The common-sense, non-scientific and anti-intellectual approach to nursing education and service can be heard in health centers by physicians and some nurses of the old culture who miss their doing-oriented nurses and practical handmaidens. Thus a struggle between the two ideological positions or sets of cultural norms regarding what makes a "good" nurse practitioner currently exists in some nursing and medical centers.

The emerging new culture of nursing which emphasizes the theoretical and scientific foundations of nursing practice is giving impetus to the profession largely by nurses who have been prepared through doctoral programs in nursing and in health-related disciplines. These research and theory leaders in nursing are providing the thrust for a new kind of nursing practice and leadership in this health field.

Uniformity and Diversity

In the 1930's, when nursing was endeavoring to standardize its clinical practices and educational programs, the norms of uniformity and conformity seemed to dominate the field. One of the forces that led to conformity was the famous 1937 Curriculum Guide which was actually intended to offer teachers of nursing some guidelines for upgrading and improving the quality of teaching in schools of nursing. In the course of time, this Guide and selected other nursing publications had the unintended impact of routinizing and standardizing content and teaching approaches in nursing schools across the country. Accordingly, nursing practice became standardized and less imaginative.

Interestingly, as nurses of the traditional culture became increasingly disposed to conformity in nursing practice and teaching, they also appeared to outsiders to act and dress alike. Strangers to nursing have interesting accounts to show the uniformity in nurses' behavior and even in their appearance. One leader in nursing vividly recalls the following incident which highlights the latter point. In the 1940's and at a nursing convention held in a moderately large city in the west, a nursing leader happened to be standing with two non-nurses in the lobby of the hotel prior to the nurses' arrival at the convention center. The nursing leader commented to the two non-nurse strangers, "I am supposed to meet two nurses here whom I have never met before. I am wondering how I will recognize them." One of the non-nurse strangers quickly replied, "That should not be difficult, but maybe it is because you're a nurse. We can always tell nurses by three facts, namely, 1) they always travel and move together with their own nursing group, 2) they always talk about their professional work and "their patients," and 3) they are generally not well dressed and usually wear dark-colored dresses." This was the perceptive and descriptive account by a non-nurse informant in the 1940's who had made repeated observations of nurses over a span of time. Although the clustering of nurses in groups continues today, nurses are becoming smartly and colorfully fashioned in their dress styles and appearances. As a result of their educational and broad social experiences, they can now talk about subjects other than nursing and "their patients." The public image of nursing is gradually changing from the traditional "bedpan servant" to an intellectual nurse with diverse skills and talents.

There has been a tendency for nurses in education and service settings to hold dissimilar views about nursing practice and education; however, their views are becoming more similar lately. By and large, uniformity in general nursing trends, issues, and problems tends to follow the thinking of a few cultural heroines in nursing today. Highly divergent and counter viewpoints are somewhat rare in the nursing field. This may be a carry-over from the old culture and a fear of being rejected by their own nursing professional group if they maintain or take a controversial stance. It is also interesting to note that in most of the professional nursing journals, highly controversial articles are seldom found; instead one finds articles which have a high probability of being fully accepted by the majority of their readers. Moreover, much of the content of these articles has been known to most nurses long before published, and so they already feel comfortable with the information. In schools of nursing, one can generally identify uniformity in faculty members' thinking which often follows that of the dominant leader(s) in the school. Even in some collegiate schools diversity of thinking and action are discouraged as they might "rock the boat too much" or cause disharmony and conflict in the school's operaion. The increasing demand by a growing number of innovative thinkers and leaders in nursing are producing pressure for traditional leaders to permit more divergent views and freedom of thinking in schools of nursing and pracice centers. There are many signs that diversity of viewpoints of young nursing leaders must be accommodated or the profession may lose imaginative and resourceful faculty. It is, indeed, a challenge to see how these young emerging leaders will be utilized in schools of nursing in the future. In a similar manner, health care systems which have been traditionally routinized and uniform in thought and practice need to be changed to accomodate the fresh and different views of an emerging new group of nurse clinicians.

Practicality and High Idealism

In the traditional culture of nursing, the terms, "practical," "intuitive," and "common-sense" were frequently used to characterize a "good" nurse and "good" nursing care practices. Many nurses claimed that their "common-sense" attitude and approach to patients was the principal means that helped them to give good nursing care. The nurse of the traditional culture was praised and rewarded for being "down-to-earth" and "practical." Currently, there is a gradual shift occurring away from this cultural norm in nursing and nurses are becoming scientific, theoretical and rationalistic." Nurses of the new culture assert that nurses should be scientific in their approach and base their nursing care practices upon theoretical and scientific principles. They believe nursing practices should focus upon specific nurse-patient problems and should be systematically studied by the collection of empirical data related to the problem. They deplore the common-sense and intuitive approach to nursing practice and claim that nursing is or should be a "learned and scientific" professional field.

Still another cultural feature can be identified in nurses of the new culture in that they appear to be highly idealistic and intellectual in their ways of looking at health problems. Nurses of the old culture feel that the "new nurses" are not close to the "realities of life situations and seem removed from the concrete problems of nursing." They contend that idealism, over-intellectualism, and some lack of emotional feeling for life situations characterize nurses of the new culture. From the author's experiences, it seems that the current idealism and intellectualism noted in nursing is a result of strong goal-achievement and the desire of nurses of the new culture to make nursing a truly scientific, intellectual, and automous discipline. The current behavior might also be explained as a reaction-formation mechanism to break away from the old cultural norms of conformity and nonscientifism to that of diversity of thought and the use of scientific research methods to study nursing.

Focus of Care

In the traditional culture of nursing practice, it was clear that the primary focus of nursing was on the physical needs of patients—keeping the patient clean, fed, protected, and warm. The expected role of the nurse in the past was to be a direct assistant to the physician, to administer an array of medicines and treatments to patients, and to provide for a patient's physical comfort. Gradually, the nurse began to focus upon the psychological needs of patients. This development occurred as a result of the impact of Adler's psychological approach to patients, the evolving psychosomatic field of study, and the psychodynamic theory of patient behavior. Considerable emphasis was given in the past to the disease or pathological state of the patient and there was limited concern for the patient who came from a certain cultural background having special life experiences.

With the present emerging new culture of nursing, social factors related to the patient's behavior are being increasingly considered with greater specification of ideas than found in the traditional culture of nursing. Most recently, cultural and other anthropological concepts have begun to make their way into the field and are providing new insights about health problems and needs of people from different communities. Both the anthropological and sociological concepts of health and illness are providing new frameworks for health practices.[5]

Role Behavior

In the traditional culture of nursing, nurses were expected to maintain primarily an *expressive-giving role* to many patients, that is they were expected to be nurturant, tender, loving, sympathetic, compassionate, protective, and giving to patients. This expressive-giving care was administered by most nurses in a casual and effective way and largely through physical ministrations to patients. Nurses believed that their warm and spontaneous maternal "instincts" were constantly in operation and could play a significant role in helping patients.

Later, as nurses became more involved with the technologies of nursing and with the pressure to care for a number of patients, many of the expressive attributes of nursing seemed to wane and become more *instrumental*. As nursing service personnel became more involved in managerial, supervisory, and administrative tasks, they became more instrumental in their thoughts and actions. Instrumental role behavior as an early sign of the new culture of nursing is concerned with explicit goals and with ideas and practices related to means toward certain goals. Nurses who are instrumentally oriented, work toward explicitly defined objectives in giving patient care. This approach has changed the character of nursing practice for there is more focus upon the various means to achieve different kinds of nursing care goals and ways to efficiently and effectively achieve such goals. With the emphasis upon instrumental role behavior, some of the direct patient care activities that traditionally belonged to the professional nurse became delegated to auxiliary nursing personnel and the nurse functioned largely in a supervisory or administrative role. For a while the supervisory duties of the nurse seemed desirable; however, it soon became evident that the professional nurse was really not satisfied in removing herself from giving direct care to patients. During the past decade, the role of the clinical specialist (which first began in psychiatric nursing in 1955) emerged, in which the nurse was prepared to function as an expert practitioner in the direct care of patients. This clinical specialist who is prepared through a graduate program on the master's level combines both *expressive* and *instrumental* role behavior to give comprehensive care to patients. It has been fascinating to see the changes in the nurse's use of expressive and instrumental role-taking with patients and how they seem to currently be merging together. It is of interest to note that male nurses have generally taken instrumental roles in the past and are frequently involved in administrative nursing services in which they provide indirect services to patients or clients; however, lately some male nurses are interested in the expressive components of nursing practice.

Psychiatric nurse clinicians tend to emphasize expressive role behaviors in therapeutic interventions with patients and families; whereas nurses in other fields tend to give equal emphasis to both expressive and instrumental role as they work with people. Female nurses in administrative roles try to combine both role behaviors; however at times it seems most difficult to maintain a happy balance of them and nurse administrators tend to become more instrumental than expressive in their activities. In our Anglo-American culture, one generally finds that patients expect nurses to be empathetic, comforting, nurturant, and giving persons and to use these expressive role behaviors in patient care. It will be of interest to see if nurses retain the expressive role behavior with people as administrative and technological tasks increase and as they become involved in managerial and political activities related to providing new kinds of health care nursing services. Whether expressive and administrative role behaviors can be successfully combined in giving nursing care is both a professional challenge and a problem for nurses. It is currently an implicit desired norm of the new culture of nursing.

Symbolic Crutches

An interesting feature of both the traditional and new cultures of nursing is the way nurses rely upon symbolic objects as important media to help patients. Traditionally, the cap, uniform, pin, white hose, and white shoes were symbolic referents to communicate immediately to the patient that the person approaching him was a nurse. But there were also other physical symbols and crutches used by nurses to relate to patients. For example, the public health nurse had several objects such as the black bag (with all its "magical" objects inside), the folded papers, the pin, and a special uniform. Often these external symbols served as important media to let the patient know immediately that a professional person was providing health service to him.

With the new culture of nursing, many of these symbolic media are not being used or relied upon so heavily as in the past to help the patient. In fact, perceptive nurses are questioning the purpose of these external symbols and their function as the nurse gives patient care. Instead, nurses are using their professional skills and themselves as the primary and important means to help people. For some nurses, it has been a drastic shift to rely upon maintaining a therapeutic relationship with a patient without depending so much on external symbols such as the uniform, cap, and black bag. Since interpersonal skills are held to be the medium for providing therapeutic care to patients, the traditional nurse has had to learn the scientific principles and techniques for establishing and maintaining effective relationships with her clients. This new emphasis has not only been a struggle for some nurses, it has revealed much fascinating data about the uses and functions of symbolic objects as crutches to nursing practices. Still today, nurses and the public depend upon the use of a set of symbolic referents to relate to one another.

Personality Attributes and "Professionalism"

In the traditional nursing culture, nurses were socialized to be dignified, self-controlled, and passive, and to maintain harmony in the system. Argyris' study demonstrated the existence of these dominant qualities and also found that nurses generally were characterized by the desire to be needed by others.[6] The nurse of the past had a noteworthy ability to endure strong pressures and demands and to remain self-controlled under such stresses. Nurses of the traditional culture tried to maintain peace and harmony in the system and to accept a wide variety of behavior. They were quick to resolve problems in a peaceful way and to withstand personal insults. Amazingly in the past, nurses were taught to control their personal feelings to patients, to their families, or to staff and to "maintain a professional attitude." Moreover, they were generally advised that it was not "professional" to discuss their home background, religious matters (except in religious schools and hospitals), politics, or any emotionally-laden topic with patients. The implicit culture norm was that talking about such topics would make the patient uncomfortable and possibly precipitate or aggrevate an acute illness state. The nurse's passivity was revealed by her willingness to have others initiate activities or action. Thus the nurse of the past was socialized to be a highly self-controlled and competent person with patients and to be deferent and humble to those in a superior role. Most important, the nurse was never to reveal her emotional feelings to patients nor to speak unduly open in her viewpoints to others.

Traditional "professionalism" was often characterized by the nurse who spoke in a quiet manner and controlled herself. Seldom did she argue or talk loudly to others in public and patient settings. Even when the nurse was "off duty," she was expected to maintain a professional attitude. Flirtatious behavior, rowdiness, hyperactivity, or gang-like behavior was questionable demeanor for a professional nurse. The quiet, conforming student who followed the rules of the school and seldom talked loudly or argued with others was rewarded by her superiors. Seldom did nurses smoke or drink liquor as this would have been viewed as a smudge in their character. Her manner has been frequently described by her associates as a person who "rolled with the punches" in responding to and handling difficult stresses and problems of the profession. "Stability in thought, action, and responsibility with a high commitment to her professional work" describes most nurses of the traditional culture of nursing.

The above picture of the traditional nurse has changed, or is in the process of changing within the new culture of nursing. In contrast, nurses are expected by the current ideal norms to be highly self-expressive, limitedly self-controlled, moderately aggressive, challenging to others, and desirous of changes. In classroom and clinical settings, the nurse is encouraged to be vocal about her observations and ideas related to patient care and clinical situations. She is eager for changing conditions in a relatively short period of time and becomes easily frustrated and/or discouraged if change does not take place quickly. The nurse of the emerging culture appears to like situations loosely controlled and not to have them too highly organized or structured. The nurse of the new culture is candid to say that she does not have all the answers to health or life situations and is fairly comfortable with not knowing everything about every situation. Generally the nurse is open and willing to "say it as it is" or "to tell it as it is" without hiding the facts about a situation. Most important, the nurse is expected to use her own personality attributes to the fullest extent in helping people. The psychiatric nursing expectation of "the use of self" is becoming an explicit professional norm which nurses are expected to be comfortable with today. The nurse of the new culture does not desire to maintain a professional attitude when "off duty." Instead, she is often loud, boisterous, flirtatious, hyperactive, prankish, and subject to gang-like behavior in an apartment or dormitory. In classroom situations, collegiate nurses are especially vocal about their own views of a situation and several are willing and capable of pursuing a heated argument with the teacher about a subject of special interest to the student. A deferent and passive attitude in the student-teacher situation in college settings seems to be vanishing.

In the clinical situation, the nurse is not expected to unduly conceal her emotions from patients, nor to respond to patients in a highly controlled manner. Instead, the nurse is taught to be natural and frank in expressing her feelings to patients and staff. Expression of one's feelings to others indicates that nurses are viable and expressive. Collegiate students are expected to talk to patients and staff on a variety of human interest topics. Their range of knowledge and versatility in changing subject topics is noteworthy. It is common to hear this young nurse discuss religious views, politics, business management, horticulture, art, music, and sundry other topics with patients.

Interestingly, the nurse of the new culture is currently being viewed as a person who is not exhibiting a long period of commitment to a professional position. A sense of deep commitment to one's professional work and the carrying forth of assigned responsibilities in a dependable and reliable manner over a fairly long period of time are not generally viewed to characterize the nurse of the new culture. In contrast with the past, the nurse of today appears restless and constantly ready for changes and she does change positions frequently. She has a broad view of societal problems, life situations, and the world of reality which she uses in nursing situations as well as in non-nursing situations. Her professional work appears as a temporary part of her life endeavors, and so a deep commitment to nursing is less apparent. It is important to emphasize that only recently have many of the qualities of the new culture begun to become apparent and especially in collegiate schools of nursing. It will be interesting to see if these qualities are sustained and further developed.

In both the old and new culture of nursing, one still finds many major decisions and evaluations being made on data largely of a personalized nature rather than using more objective and nonpersonalized data. For example, factual data presented in a project report may be unconsciously disregarded in committee evaluations for personal evaluations regarding who the person is that submitted the report, her home school or university, and sketchy personal accounts about the project director. Some members of the profession are gradually becoming aware of this problem and are making efforts to handle evaluations and major decisions in a more scientific manner and less personalized way.

Presenting some of the major features of the culture of nursing has value in helping nurses become aware of the major professional configurations which characterize the field of nursing. Undoubtedly the reader may have placed herself as belonging to the old or new culture or she may realize that she has attributes and qualities of both cultures. It is clear that the two cultures of nursing exist and there are many historical and professional reasons which support their existence. There is, indeed, evidence that a rapid acculturation process is occurring with nurses moving more and more to the features of the new culture of nursing. However, there are features of the traditional culture which professional members of this culture are eager to retain, such as attitudes of responsibility, dependability, and stability. It will be interesting to see what attributes of the two cultures are retained. Will the new culture come fully into existence, or will an entirely different culture of nursing emerge in the future?

FOOTNOTES

[1] In this chapter, the author will speak of the culture of nursing as a shorthand way of referring to the subculture of nursing.

[2] David Reisman, *The Lonely Crowd*, New Haven, Connecticut: Yale University Press, 1950.

[3] Genevieve Rogge Meyer, *Tenderness and Technique: Nursing Values in*

Transition, Los Angeles: University of California Institute of Industrial Relations, 1960, pp. 1-11.

[4] I. M. Stewart, *The Education of Nurses*, New York: Macmillan, 1947.

[5] Benjamin Paul, Editor, *Health, Culture and Community: Case Studies of Public Relations to Health Programs*, New York: Russell Sage Foundation, 1955.

[6] C. Argyris, *Diagnosing Human Relations in Organizations: A Case Study of a Hospital*, New Haven Connecticut: Labor and Management Center, Yale University, 1956.

6 Cultural Differences between Patient and Staff, and Their Influence on Patient Care

Understanding Cultural Differences: The Key to Success

Man as a cultural and social being has many needs which are usually fulfilled by cultural norms and interaction with others. Becoming aware of differences in cultural values, norms, and practices is necessary if one wishes to communicate, work, and enjoy life with other people. Professional health workers who deal intimately with people in health and illness states must learn about differences of cultural groups and seek ways to become alert to such differences in giving patient care.

In the past, there has been a tendency for health personnal to label patients "impossible," "difficult," or "uncooperative" when they found it was difficult to understand a patient's behavior. This approach has not been too effective because often it leads to staff isolation of the patient and a tendency for the staff to reduce their efforts to understand the patient. The use of such behavioral labels gives important clues to cultural differences between patients and staff and should lead to a study and analysis of patient and staff interrelationships and behavior. The "difficult" or "uncooperative" patient may well be encountering problems which are of a cultural or social nature and problems which the nursing staff do not understand. The nurse, too may be exhibiting behavior that disturbs the patient. Indeed, these factors need to be identified and dealt with if the staff desires to affect a successful program of nursing care. Armed with the analysis of the situation, the nurse can offer rational, intelligent, and empathetic care regarding cultural needs of patients. In this chapter, the author will focus upon cultural differences between the patient and the staff, and examine how these differences influence the patient. It is the author's belief that marked cultural differences between the patient and the staff can have both positive and negative consequences, but the key to success is to understand cultural differences among patients and between patients and staff.

As one might suspect, marked differences in cultural backgrounds of the patient and staff may be a source of considerable distrust, social distance, curiosity, and alienation. These behaviors often become apparent as one observes and studies closely an interaction process between two strangers, or between persons who become aware that they have differences in ways of living and thinking. Generally, there are communication clues between people which reveal interpersonal tensions related to cultural differences in communication and in general behavior patterns. If health personnel are not alert to the role of cultural factors in communication and in ongoing relationships, they may miss many cues about the nature and source of the difficulty. In staff and team conferences the sociocultural factors influencing relationship patterns are frequently not discussed or used specifically in planning care in the same manner as psychophysiological factors of patient care.

Before further pursuing the chapter topic, several relevant questions can be asked as a guide to the discussion of cultural factors and staff-patient behavior: (1) How do cultural background differences between the patient and the staff facilitate or hinder the care and treatment process? (2) Is it more helpful if patients and staff have a similar cultural background or a dissimilar cultural background? (3) How can one therapeutically help a patient if his cultural background differs considerably from the nurse who works directly with him? (4) What do we know about patients' behavior when the patient experiences "culturally different kinds of stresses" in nursing situations? (5) What are some of the recurrent problems that exist in health systems because of differences in cultural backgrounds between staff and patients? (6) What studies should be made to resolve problems related to culture differences and their impact on patients? At the present time there is a paucity of research studies which answer any of these questions. And yet the questions seem so relevant today and so basic to quality patient care. Let us briefly consider some possible explanations of why these questions have not been given attention in the past.

Reasons for the Neglect of Key Questions

The first and most obvious reason is that health personnel are only recently becoming aware of the role of cultural factors in health care, and especially the nursing staff. Even if some nurses showed an interest in exploring how cultural factors affect patient care, they may have had limited support or encouragement from others in studying this aspect of patient care. Or, if the nurse felt free to examine cultural factors related to patient care, she may have felt reluctant to pursue the study, fearing this might be a taboo area of study for nurses. Some nurses may have been instructed in their educational program that one does not talk with patients about intimate data such as cultural background factors. This state of affairs may exist where nurses are encouraged not to discuss any religious, social, political, and cultural factors related to patients and families. There is evidence that this taboo exists today as some nurses believe that intimate conversation with patients cannot be pursued as it leads to emotionally-laden content which the nurse cannot handle effectively. Indeed, the nurse who assumes this belief would naturally avoid looking at cultural background factors in the patient-staff relationships. With the encouraging trend of nurses receiving a combined professional and liberal arts education in collegiate institutions, nurses are beginning to show signs of being more at ease in exploring and dealing with their own sociocultural backgrounds and that of the patient and staff.

Of course, there are some nurses who have expressed concern about working with a patient whose cultural background was different from hers; however, she may have been at a loss knowing how best to help the patient because of her limited knowledge about anthropology. Or, if the nurse had some knowledge about the patient's cultural heritage, she might have relinquished the idea of a culturally-tailored nursing care plan because of a lack of confidence in what she was doing. Often what happens in this situation is that the nurse ends up treating the patient the same way that she cares for all patients. Basic knowledge deficits might easily account for the lack of interest in studying and making specific nursing care plans for a patient from another culture.

Our American cultural value of democracy and the high emphases upon egalitarianism might well be another deciding factor that has led the nurse not to study or help the patient in a specific cultural way. In this instance, the nurse would feel she is violating an American democratic principle by focusing on a particular patient. Or, if she did direct her attention to a particular patient, she might have developed feelings of guilt and doubt because she had broken a cultural norm in nursing, namely, spending too much time, attention, and care on one patient when the implicit norm is to give equal consideration to all patients on her unit. This nurse might also be subject to peer group (and supervisor) disapproval, criticism, and social alienation. Conflicts between the prescribed American cultural and nursing norms can curtail the nurse's desire to work with a patient from a different culture and to implement specific nursing care plans that include cultural factors.

Finally, if the nurse did feel a genuine interest in helping a patient whose cultural background was similar to hers, she might have quickly dismissed the idea because of negative feelings and unresolved problems related to her own cultural background, self-identity, and self-understanding. Some nurses from a particular culture carry with them a negative feeling about their cultural origin, and they try to suppress or deny their own cultural identity. To work with a patient who would activate one's own unresolved feelings would be difficult. This situation could be especially aggravating to nurses from particular cultural groups which are currently looked down upon by other cultural and class-oriented groups. Sometimes, people who have deep feelings of anger and resentment toward members of their own cultural groups live as if they belonged to another cultural group. If the nurse has such strong feelings about her own cultural identity and background, she should not be forced or unduly persuaded to help patients whose backgrounds are similar to hers. There are, however, some nurses who are slightly aware of such feelings and have requested to work with patients if they can have supervision from qualified nurse-anthropologists. This is a healthy and positive approach to resolve a nursing care problem.

Let us now consider some realistic patient-staff situations in order to help us understand some of the positive and negative effects that cultural factors can have on patient-staff relationships. The situations presented here are ones which were known personally to the author, her staff colleagues, and her students.

Patient-Staff Study Situations

Study One: German-American Patient. A 60-year-old German-American patient was in a state psychiatric hospital for ten years. He was viewed by the staff as an agitated, withdrawn, and depressed patient who would probably never leave the hospital. At the age of 25 years, Mr. G. and his German wife came to the United States from his homeland of Germany, and settled in a small German community in Pennsylvania where he worked hard to become a successful baker. Mr. G. had one son who was married and lived in a nearby state. The patient had never learned to speak English except for a few common greetings and idiomatic expressions.

During the first eight years that Mr. G. was in the psychiatric hospital, he remained quietly on a "back ward," except for periodic episodes of talking loudly and angrily in German to the staff and pacing rapidly back and forth in the ward hallways. Since the majority of the staff were Anglo-American, none of them understood German. They did not know what the patient was saying in German, but they knew he was angry. The staff made an initial attempt to reduce his loud talking and ward pacing by talking in English to him, but when this did not yield a positive response they would place him in a "quiet room" until he relinquished the noisy behavior. Chemical sedation was also a common method used to reduce Mr. G.'s aggressive and hyperactive behavior. This was the major behavioral theme of Mr. G. and the usual staff response to him. Through time, the staff took care of Mr. G.'s basic physical needs and did not show an interest in the past background of Mr. G.

During the eighth year of Mr. G.'s hospitalization, a clinical specialist in psychiatric nursing began working on Mr. G.'s ward. Miss Meyer, the nurse, was a third generation German-American whose parents spoke German and lived in many ways like their German ancestors in Europe. Miss Meyer, however, had not spoken German since she was ten years of age, but she understood some German expressions and could say a few German greetings. Shortly after this nurse was on the ward, she became interested in Mr. G. and his behavior. She could not specify why she was interested in Mr. G., but "something drew her closer to this patient." The first time Miss Meyer spoke to Mr. G. with a common German greeting, the patient was very surprised and began to talk rapidly to the nurse using his hands to add expression to his words. Miss Meyer could not understand all that he was saying, but she listened attentively to him by sitting silently and focusing her eyes on him. In subsequent encounters, she repeated this behavior. Frequently, she found him sitting in a certain chair and alone. Mr. G. responded cautiously, but warmly to the interest and attention shown to him by Miss Meyer. Whenever they spent time together, Mr. G. showed an eagerness to talk to her. Miss Meyer was frustrated because she could not understand everything the patient said to her. She did, however, get snatches which helped her know the patient's feelings of loneliness and anger. One day, Miss Meyer decided to learn German from her parents and with the aid of German conversation books. Her parents, who were proud of their German heritage, were delighted to know that their daughter was taking an interest in German, and so they helped her considerably. Miss Meyer was an apt student and was quick to learn the language she knew as a child. She was always eager "to practice" her German with Mr. G., which delighted him immeasurably.

The turning point in Mr. G.'s long illness and hospitalization seemed to occur with Miss Meyer's interest in him, and especially since she was able to talk with him in his native language. There was a noticeable change in his behavior. Mr. G. seemed to see and experience a new world of hope, trust, and non-alienation. Bonds of interest, mutual concern, warmth, and friendliness between the patient and nurse became apparent. It seemed as if the patient had long experienced his own world of illness, and now he was sharing this world with someone else who was interested in it. Mr. G.'s feelings of anger and despair diminished, and the nurse discovered a kind and special person. Knowledge of the language was one of the crucial means to reach the patient, and Miss Meyer accepted this challenge. Knowing the patient's language helped considerably to reduce the barrier between Mr. G.'s intrapsychic and interpersonal worlds. Furthermore, it helped the other staff members to become interested in the patient—for the first time in many years.

In due time, Miss Meyer was able to get Mr. G. to join a small group of male patients in playing shuffleboard and cards after many years of being a "loner" in social activities. The patient gradually began to enjoy the companionship of other patients and the staff, with Miss Meyer serving as his interpreter and agent in facilitating social interaction. One day, Miss Meyer learned from Mr. G. that, among other things, he had been a good baker—a fact which none of the staff knew. In the course of discussing Mr. G.'s culinary interests, the nurse observed that he became noticeably excited and "alive." His eyes sparkled and he made gestures with his hands showing the way he made bread many years ago. It was clear from his talk and mannerisms that the patient's worth, self-esteem, and pride increased whenever he talked about his old occupation. He became so involved in reliving this experience that his behavior seemed extremely rational and appropriate.

Miss Meyer, a very perceptive nurse, noticed that the patient's self esteem had improved noticeably and he was rediscovering himself as a person who had been highly respected in the past for his bread-making. She decided to ask Mr. G. if he would like to make a batch of bread some day. Mr. G. stared at her and said, "No . . . I don't think I can. It has been such a long time since I made any bread. I don't know the recipe. I can't do it." They talked more about the recipe and the steps in making his favorite bread. Soon, Mr. G. was able to recall the recipe and demonstrated with his hands how he made bread. One day he said, "I think I can make bread, but I have always made large batches of bread for many people." Miss Meyer then checked the feasibility of having Mr. G. make a large batch of bread for the institution. The chief cook was skeptical about the patient's ability to make bread and the possible loss of costly bread materials if the recipe failed. However, the plans were finalized and Mr. G. pursued the task of making a large batch of bread. Again, he became so enthusiastic in the task that it was heart-warming to watch him. He made a successful and delicious batch of homemade bread. The aroma from his cooking of the bread permeated the building, and patients and staff all enjoyed his fine bread. The patient was surprised and proud of his achievement, and the staff were equally amazed to see what Mr. G. was able to do after so many years of inactivity in the hospital. This positive experience had a great influence on changing Mr. G.'s behavior and also the course of his hospitalization. Mr. G. seemed to be a different person who trusted and talked to others. His anger had abated, and he was more congenial and sociable. He sang German songs for the other patients and showed more interest in what patients were doing and saying. Eight months after Miss Meyer had begun nursing therapy with Mr. G., he was dismissed from the hospital and returned to his old German-American community. He was encouraged to work part-time in a bakery, and he followed through on this suggestion, enjoying the work considerably.

This is an actual account of what happened to Mr. G. The role of the nurse in discovering the patient through an understanding of his cultural background and by learning the patient's language were extremely important factors in bringing Mr. G. to a dramatic and successful recovery. To recapitulate, Miss Meyer was quick to note how important it was to know the patient through his native language and she was willing to meet the challenge by learning German. Through his own language, Miss Meyer discovered Mr. G. emotionally, culturally, and socially. It became clear that the patient's German background had remained important to him, serving as a guide to his daily way of life since he came from Germany more than forty years ago. The cultural ties from his native land to his German-American community had been firmly retained and reinforced. This patient-study helps the nurse realize that one's cultural values remain an active and significant part of one's life even when one moves to another environment and lives their. How lonely and displaced Mr. G. must have been for many years on a psychiatric back ward, until a sensitive and interested nurse discovered the patient's own world! Retrospectively, one wonders if Mr. G. would have ever been dismissed from the hospital had Miss Meyer not come on the ward and helped him. What would have happened to him?

Miss Meyer learned many things about Mr. G. in her on-going relationship with him. She learned that Mr. G.'s wife had always brought her husband baked foods until she died twelve years ago, at which time Mr. G. became markedly depressed. Miss Meyer realized that she was perceived by Mr. G. as his wife—a woman who was interested in him and his work. Mr. G. had always been an industrious man, and his wife was quick to praise him. By speaking German to Mr. G., the nurse conveyed not only a genuine interest in the patient and his cultural background, but also discovered Mr. G.'s feelings of loneliness, distrust, and anger. Through the language, Mr. G. was able to disclose his long pent-up feelings toward the staff, life in general, and the fact that he had lost his wife. It was amazing to see Mr. G.'s patterned behavior of social alienation and loneliness changed to one of social enjoyment with others. Although Miss Meyer might have been able to relate with the patient on an empathetic non-verbal level, still one wonders if this form of communication would have been satisfying to him, for Mr. G. loved to talk and express his feelings. Verbal communication seemed to increase Mr. G.'s self-confidence, hope, and self-esteem. The patient spent many days talking with the nurse about his sad feelings when his wife died. Miss Meyer is to be commended for her willingness to learn the German language and to remain with the patient until he found himself again. The skills of this psychiatric nurse specialist were gained in a master's degree program in psychiatric nursing, and so she was fully aware of the process of nursing therapy. In addition, Miss Meyer was interested in cultural factors influencing psychiatric behavior and pursued her interests with encouragement from a nurse-anthropologist in another city.

Study Two: Italian-American Child. Mario was a four-year-old child of Italian-American descent who was brought to the hospital for surgical repair of a congenital heart defect. After several months of serious family discussions, Mario's parents and grandparents had decided to have Mario's heart defect corrected. It was, however, a most difficult decision because the family was skeptical of surgery and the kind of care their child would receive on a busy hospital ward.

Cultural factors played a significant part in the parents' consent to the surgery and in the plans for the child's care after surgery. The parents had consented to have the surgery only after an Italian-American heart surgeon had discussed the surgery with them and had agreed to do the surgery. It had been a great relief to talk to a physician who had a cultural background similar to their own. In addition, Mario's parents wanted "their own Italian-American nurse" to care for their son. She was a nurse whom the family had known for several years. Miss Lanzo, the nurse, was willing to work with the family and take care of their son from eight in the morning until six in the evening, and then the nurse had two other nurses whom she knew very well to care for Mario during the remaining hours. This was comforting and reassuring to Mario's parents. They felt that their son would be in the hands of persons who would understand him because they could relate to these Italian-American professional personnel.

Specific cultural norms were at work in this situation. Mario was the only son in the family and, traditionally, Italian males are loved and wanted since they are important cultural carriers of the family heritage. Also, there is usually a strong bond between an Italian-American mother and her son—a bond of devotion, love, and closeness. Mario's mother wanted to be sure that her care-taking responsibilities were being performed by a reliable mother substitute—her Italian-American nurse friend. Mario's mother depended upon this nurse to provide comfort, care, and security that she herself usually gave her son and to blend her professional skills with this motherly care as characterized by the Italian culture. The Italian father, too, shared in the over-all plans for the son and showed a protective and fatherly interest in him. So the Italian surgeon was viewed as the symbolic referent for the father's responsibilities and concerns. In sum, one finds a fascinating, substitute family situation being established by the professional personnel in order to provide care to a child whom the Italian-American family dearly loved and cherished. These plans were carefully thought about before Mario was brought to the hospital.

Mario and his parents were born in the United States; however, his paternal grandparents were born in Italy and had been living in the U.S. for only four years. The grandparents (from both descent lines) were closely aligned to Mario's family, and they lived as one large extended family. Whenever this extended family faced a crisis, all members became strongly united and empathetically felt the stress of the person under undue stress.

Fortunately, Mario's surgery and recovery were successful. There were many factors contributing to the success. Mario's parents and paternal grandparents came every morning and evening to be with Mario in his hospital room. They talked, laughed, and played with Mario in their culturally defined ways, and Mario responded to them in his physically handicapped, but warm and affectionate manner. Miss Lanzo, the Italian-American nurse, naturally and beautifully combined her cultural background behavior with her professional skills to give Mario the best care possible; moreover, one could note how much she enjoyed the challenge and opportunity to be a good Italian-American mother surrogate and nurse to Mario. The heart surgeon also seemed comfortable combining his cultural and professional skills to reassure the family members about every phase of the surgery and the post-surgery treatment of the child. Thus the Italian-American nurse and the surgeon were invaluable cultural personnel to the family, and they were able to help the other staff members on the service understand and help the Italian-American family. All members of the "cultural team" spoke Italian and English, and it was interesting to observe that under extreme stress periods and while discussing highly confidential material the family and clinic team spoke Italian, but that when common public matters were being discussed, English was spoken. Anthropologists have noted, in their study of people who are bilingual, that information which is private and important to a cultural group tends to be revealed only in the native language.

Study Three: Spanish-Speaking Patient Group. A small group of twelve Spanish-speaking male and female patients were receiving treatment in a psychiatric hospital located in the southern Rocky Mountain region. The majority of the patients had been in the hospital for approximately three months. Although most of the patients were bilingual, speaking both Spanish and English, they preferred to speak Spanish. These patients were receiving milieu and group therapy.

An Anglo-American psychiatrist had been working with a group of patients who were from diverse cultural backgrounds; he noticed that the group sessions had not been going well because most of the patients found it difficult to communicate with one another, and that he was having particular difficulty communicating with the Spanish-American patients. The melange of patients from different cultural and linguistic backgrounds made it difficult for the patients to communicate with one another about their problems and feelings. Of most importance, the patients did not seem to want to discuss their personal problems with "strangers." Approximately one-half of the patients in the group were Spanish-Americans and Mexican-Americans, and they were the most non-communicative members of the group. The problem of how best to work with them had been discussed in several staff meetings.

While the Spanish-speaking patients had been in group therapy, they had daily sought out two nursing assistants who spoke Spanish and were of their same cultural background. The Spanish-speaking patients talked to the assistants about their dislike of being in the group sessions and the reasons why they objected. These patients were extremely reluctant to discuss their "own family problems with strangers;" however, they felt obligated to attend the group meetings since it was "ordered" for them. In addition, these patients found it very difficult to understand the problems of other patients, as they could not perceive these problems from their cultural framework, and could not understand the purpose of the group meetings. As these Spanish-speaking patients continued to talk each day about their problems in being in the group, a spontaneous group formed on the ward and the two Spanish-speaking nursing assistants were being placed as the natural leaders for the group sessions. This practice was viewed as a promising situation, and the assistants were supervised by a skilled psychiatric nursing clinician. The nursing assistants took the leadership role reluctantly; however, with encouragement and supervision, they performed the task very well.

It was amazing to observe how these Spanish-speaking patients responded to one another in "their own" group sessions. They were quite comfortable in talking about their concerns with one another and with two nursing assistants who were from the same cultural background as they were. During the group sessions, the Spanish-speaking patients talked about their feelings about their relationships with Anglo- and Afro-Americans. They also discussed "family secrets" regarding strained kinship relationships. This behavior might have been anticipated since Spanish-Americans and Mexican-Americans feel much safer if they can talk about their own family and cultural problems within a group who have similar problems. Revealing highly personal and family information to strangers, such as the non-Spanish psychiatrist or nurse, was a cultural taboo for these patients. Some patients had talked about a few of their intimate secrets to the psychiatrist, and feelings of guilt and distrust emerged as they were breaking a cultural norm. Furthermore, Spanish-Americans and

Mexican-Americans see emotional difficulties as a kind of life trial which is given to them by God, and which they must learn to accept. The Spanish-speaking patients were perplexed in the early group sessions because there was no mention about God's role in influencing the illness, and they were reluctant to talk about this with others who might not understand their beliefs about God and his role in illness. Nor did the Spanish-speaking patients see their emotional problems as something which they could resolve without God's help or intervention. These patients were also lost in understanding common psychiatric terms, such as "ambivalence" and "denial," which were used by the psychiatrist as he talked to the patients in the group sessions. Other concerns of the patients were largely cultural incidents and folk secrets which the patients did not want to share with persons who were not of the same cultural background. These factors limited the patients from using the group sessions conducted by the psychiatrist.

In the analysis of the informal and spontaneously formed group sessions conducted by the nursing assistants from the same background as the patients, the patients were much more at ease and able to talk openly to the assistants. Several reasons could be stated by the Spanish patients. To begin with they felt that they were discussing their problems and feelings with someone of their "own group" and "they understood us." Simple sentences in the patient's own vernacular helped considerably, as they were sure that what they said in Spanish would be accurately understood, and so they could talk more freely than previously with the psychiatrist. Since the nursing assistants came from the same cultural background as the patients, they were most sensitive and alert to the patients' problems and were able to pursue the problems in their familiar cultural context. Fortunately, the nursing assistants were comfortable with their own cultural heritage and drew substantially upon it to help the group of patients. These Spanish-speaking patients finally did have a successful group experience, and much of the success was due to the genuine interest in and excellent working relationships with people from their own cultural background. The psychiatric nurse was able to help the assistants make the experience as profitable as possible. She did not participate in the group session but she learned much from her supervisory sessions with the assistants.

The above actual patient study situations reveal that there are a number of positive benefits from helping patients who have similar backgrounds as that of the nurse. Some of these positive features need to be summarized here. Staff and patients with similar cultural beliefs and a similar way of life tend to identify quite readily with one another. Language is an important cultural tie which helps two strangers communicate and share their feelings. Perhaps there has not traditionally been enough emphasis in nursing upon language and its important function in helping to express feelings of empathy, trust, and identification. Since language is the important means for initiating relationships with strangers and for building reciprocal interests, one should not underestimate the importance of communicating with patients in their native language. Staff who cannot speak the native language of the patient may encounter considerable difficulty trying to help him.

Similar cultural or subcultural mannerisms, similar ways of living, and similar cultural beliefs and values are all powerful means for drawing strangers together. Knowledge of similar beliefs and practices as one shares can help one to feel safe and can provide ready-made solutions to handle recurrent life problems. In addition, similar religious practices, social life, and many other familiar life experiences help make people feel close together. In fact feelings of closeness, unity, and solidarity are often the consequence of relationships between persons who come from similar cultural backgrounds. If one observes the verbal and non-verbal forms of communication when persons from similar cultural backgrounds meet, one will note that their greeting is so warm and friendly that they could be mistaken for two lost sisters or brothers. Even the body gestures convey movement toward another. This becomes quite apparent when two persons from the same culture meet in a foreign country and their gestural and verbal communication is rapid and forceful. It is also interesting to observe what happens when two strangers meet whose cultural backgrounds are not known. There is a struggle to determine the cultural identities of the other person. Initially, there is a "feeling and testing out" process in which pleasant and safe terms of address and ritualized statements can be observed: "How are you?", "How are you feeling?", "What do you think of this weather?" These ritualized comments are usually followed by more directly probing as the two strangers continue their inquiry of one another. Personal data and then later social and cultural data are sought. Gradually, the two strangers are relieved when they find a common or shared interest which they reinforce by saying, "Yes, I have always believed in this" or "I do the same thing." A bond of similar thinking and experiences emerges, and then the relationship becomes more spontaneous and empathetic. If two strangers do not find some common cultural ties during the initial test period, they may be sufficiently curious to repeat the encounter at a time in the near future, or they may dissolve the relationship feeling there are no bonds of mutual interest to sustain it.

In the above examples, the ethnic background of the patient and nurse were similar and were valuable means for shared communication and feelings. There are occasions, however, when the use of an individual's similar cultural background may not have such positive results, and the relationship may be difficult and strained as found in the patient study which follows.

Study Four: Afro-American Patient. An Afro-American nurse, Mona, was assigned to care for an Afro-American patient called Alex in a general hospital unit. Mona, who was born and reared in the northern part of the United States, was initially uncomfortable in taking care of Alex, who was born and raised in a southern state. Mona revealed her discomfort with Alex in several ways. She would hurriedly give Alex his medications and any physical treatments, and then leave him alone until he called for something. Mona did not visit with Alex or spend any extra time with him. Her manner was curt and cold. The head nurse on the unit noticed Mona's behavior with Alex and asked about the brevity of her encounters with the patient. Mona was quick to say, "He appears like me. He belongs to my group, but I think I am different. If I spend time with Alex, the staff will think I am like him. However, I still want to give him care." Mona was experiencing real conflict and some ambivalent feelings about her own cultural identity. She talked about the disadvantages and problems of being an Afro-American, and she wanted to be "something different." But at the same time, she wanted to examine her negative feelings about her cultural heritage and to care for the patient. She did not want to get too close to the patient because she feared her negative feelings would be obvious to him. Then, too, she noted that Alex had mannerisms and language patterns which she disliked, and that his behavior was different from the Afro-Americans of the northern states.

The head nurse was most patient and understanding of Mona's problems and feelings. She realized that it was important for Mona to establish her own pace of comfortableness with Alex. Each day, she listened to Mona's feelings about herself and the patient as Mona continued her work. Mona's hurried manner and her abruptness were apparent to Alex, but he was quite tolerant of her, believing she was "busy" and therefore could not spend much time with him. Gradually, Mona realized that Alex was a human being like herself, and she found that he was a kind and warm individual whose mannerisms were not as annoying as she had found them at first. The patient, who had had an appendectomy, left the hospital on the fifth post-operative day.

Although Mona's feelings about caring for a person of her own cultural background were extremely negative, she was open and willing to learn about herself and to change her feelings. The patient was a tolerant individual who was aware of the nurse's behavior, but he was sufficiently comfortable with his own cultural identity to not be bothered by it. Mona was pleased that she remained with the patient and did not abandon him because of her initial negative feelings. She learned that there are subcultural differences between Afro-American groups in the United States and, in particular, variations between the southern and northern Afro-American's way of life.

Although other examples could be offered to show how cultural differences between the patient and staff influence patient care, the above situations convey the message. Ideally, a professional nurse should have an interest in the patient's background to help her understand him as much as possible.

Sometimes, the nurse does not know how to explore and examine cultural and social factors that influence the patient's behavior, and so she may lose an important means for establishing a therapeutic relationship with the patient. The therapeutic use of one's cultural background is a new area to explore. It is the author's position that the nurse should not be reluctant to use her cultural experiences with patients. She should learn about American subcultures, at least, and should explore ways to integrate their cultural norms into her nursing care.

7 The Use of Cultural Factors in Patient Care: Examples from Different Cultures

Recently, members of the health professions have begun to feel a need to understand people from different cultures. This need stems partly from their professional interests in helping people and partly from recent social and economic forces in our society. People from different cultural and subcultural groups in this country and elsewhere are making their identity, problems, and needs known to society-at-large. Accordingly, federal, state, and local governments are being confronted with demands and problems of different cultural groups. Professional and public groups can no longer remain indifferent to the viewpoints and needs of cultural groups. They are challenging us to understand them and to facilitate their identity and special needs into the mainstream of American life.

Actually, professional personnel should feel a sense of professional responsibility today to learn as much as they can about different cultural and subcultural groups in order to increase their therapeutic competence with patients, families, and community groups.

Ways to Gain Cultural Awareness

How can professional people become knowledgeable about different cultures and the cultural factors influencing the health care of people? How can they use this knowledge effectively in the treatment and care of sick people? Professional nurses as well as other health workers are faced today with these important questions. Perhaps the most important first step toward a resolution of these questions is that the professional person understand the concept of *cultural awareness* and develop a sensitivity to the significance of cultural factors in people's lives. To develop cultural awareness the nurse must make a *conscious and consistent* effort to study different cultural groups and their special cultural background. Taking courses in cultural and social anthropology and reading widely and thoughtfully about different cultural groups is a valuable means to develop cultural awareness. It is well known that most anthropological writings about cultural groups are usually written in a highly readable and interesting style so that the professional person will find the material fascinating and generally easy to read. In addition to formal courses and informal reading opportunities, the nurse has an excellent opportunity to understand people from different cultures by listening attentively to them as she interacts directly with them in the home, clinic, or hospital setting. The home setting is an especially ideal place to learn about cultural groups as there are many natural ways the people talk and interact with one another that are culturally defined and demonstrated in their home. Once the nurse has gained entry into the home and assumes an attitude of genuine interest in the social group, she can learn much about their cultural ways. A series of on-going participant observations with a few open-ended questions and comments can be enormously helpful to the nurse in gaining cultural knowledge and awareness.

Whatever the setting, the nurse generally has many opportunities to learn about people who have different cultural beliefs and ways of living. If she is interested in and attentive to the patient's actions and thought patterns, she can gain valuable knowledge about his culture. An open and inquiring attitude will usually enhance her possibilities of gaining new understanding about the patient. Generally, as the middle-class caucasian nurse works with a patient who belongs to a minority cultural or subcultural group, she will notice that he tends to be initially quiet, polite, conforming, and shy. This behavior often reflects a guarded or cautious response as the person is not sure what is expected of him and how the course of interaction will go. It is a "safe behavior" response for an initial encounter with a stranger; however it may not be his normal behavior pattern of interaction with non-strangers. As this person encounters unfamiliar health personnel, he believes it is wise to be initially passive and quiet as it permits him time to "size up" the staff and to present behavior which will not be too offensive or alarming to the staff. Speaking to patients from a minority group in a soft tone of voice and in a non-hurried manner often helps to put the patient at ease so he can soon "be his natural self." Aggressive, demanding, and assertive behavior on the part of professional staff often leads to patient withdrawal or silent anger so that the patient wishes he had never come for help. It is a wise and therapeutic measure to sit with the patient in a fairly silent manner and to listen to him. Sitting with the patient often makes the patient from a different cultural group feel significant and worthy of the time and attention of others. It is also advisable to spend some time with the patient's family and learn how the family and patient interact, talk together, and share ideas and concerns with one another. Making periodic visits to the patient's home generally reassures the patient and his family of the genuine and sustained interest in him and his family. Furthermore, the nurse can obtain kinds of data in the home that are usually difficult to obtain of the patient and his family in the hospital context. This is because the hospital setting often creates a strained and artificial context between patients and staff. Data collected in the hospital is often "adjustment data" in that it primarily reveals how the patient modifies or adapts himself to the hospital milieu, rather than how he normally feels in his home toward his illness and how he maintains his own health practices. As we shall learn in Chapter 10, the hospital has its own cultural norms which the patient and his family learn to adjust to with an illness experience.

Understanding Culture Factors as a Basis for Patient Care
Since culture defines *a way of life for a designated group of people*, the nurse must understand the particular way of life for a defined patient, family, or social group she (he) is trying to help. As discussed in Chapter 4, culture is a patterned way of life which has special meaning to the individual and his cultural group. Culture serves as a guide to action and beliefs as the individual meets both familiar and new life situations. Without culture, the individual would be literally a "nervous wreck," because he would have no built-in familiar ways of responding or adapting to new or strange life experiences. These built-in learned responses of people are of special importance in meeting crises or shocking situations. The nurse, therefore, needs to know the patient's cultural patterns of thinking, feeling, and acting so she can determine a therapeutic plan of care for the patient. Once the nurse has grasped the life style of the patient, she can begin to devise specific tailor-made ways to help him and to follow through and evaluate her plans. With her nursing care plan for a particular patient, she will endeavor to see the interrelationship of the patient's psychological, social, physical, and cultural needs, and try to bring them into a workable and effective plan. Of most importance, the nurse must involve the patient in planning and implementing his care plan. As the nurse involves the patient in the care plan, she identifies his familiar ways of recovering from an illness and how these cultural ways may tend to help or hinder his recovery. Certainly, the nurse must draw upon the cultural health norms of people and become aware of their impact upon the health state of the patient. She realizes that patients are generally not willing to quickly forfeit their own cultural values for temporary professional values unless the patient wants to change

his value system and believes in the rationale for the new value changes. The nurse, therefore, is aware that conflicts between the nurse's professional health norms and those of the patient may occur and must be fully recognized and dealt with in giving nursing care.

One can seriously question the rights of a particular professional group to change another person's cultural values if the client wishes to retain his values. This becomes especially crucial regarding values related to the patient's philosophy of life and death. It is the author's viewpoint that the cultural values of the patient and his family must be given full consideration, and professional staff do not have the ethical right to coerce or deliberately change a patient's cultural values for theirs unless the patient gives his consent. The deliberate and subtle ways of changing a patient's values is especially questionable with the dying patient who is in a helpless position to assert and defend his own beliefs. Sometimes the nurse unknowingly changes the patient's religious and philosophical values about life and death at a time when these beliefs are usually most comforting to him—namely at the time of death. Thus the nurse should know the patient's cultural values about life and death so that she can be a helpful person to him and not interfere with these values as he faces death. The threat of death is a crucial life experience for an individual and his cultural values have special meaning to him. Knowledge of these values can be the key to therapeutic ways of helping a dying patient or one who is experiencing the threat of death.

Knowing the patient's cultural background is also crucial to the nurse's understanding of *the role she should assume in helping* a patient and his family. It may be that a patient from a particular culture group may unconsciously want the nurse to take a cultural role such as that of a Hungarian surrogate father or a Swiss mother. If the nurse is knowledgeable about such culturally defined roles and behavior expectations, she can and will be able to determine how she and the staff can use patient role expectations in nursing care practices. Generally, different cultures have different health practitioner roles which are viewed as essential in curing or caring for a patient. Does the average nurse know what these culturally defined roles are and the behavior expectations of people in these roles? Unfortunately, many nurses may not be aware that such role-taking is important in effecting changes in the health-illness status of a patient. Anthropological literature can provide information about these roles and help the nurse consider creative approaches to role-taking in patient care. Most important, there is a *current need to link professional role behavior with that of the indigenous health practitioner's role* behavior in order to reduce cultural ambiguities and health role conflicts.

Understanding cultural factors related to patient care is also necessary if one wishes to facilitate change in the health attitudes and practices of the patient and his family. Changes in health behavior cannot be successfully achieved unless the nurse first understands what she is trying to change. If a patient does not respond well or readily to prescribed professional value changes related to health, the patient may be labeled "uncooperative," "stupid," or "resistive," but his behavior may be attributable to conflicts in health value orientations. Change in health patterns for many patients often requires some noticeable changes in their daily mode of living. The nurse must try to understand each situation from the *patient's viewpoint* and his health goals. The nurse, too, should realize that health changes in cultural values occur *within the family structure* as well as *outside the family structure*, and so she must obtain data regarding these two sources. In general, effective modifications in health practices for a patient can be assured if cultural factors are known to and understood by the health practitioner within the context of the patient's family, work, and community.

Finally, knowledge of cultural factors is important in patient care to assist in the educational process of helping other professional and non-professional staff members to become aware of cultural factors and to include these factors in patient care and staff relationships. Since many staff members are recently becoming sensitive to the importance of culture factors, the nurse, through her direct contact with patients and families, can casually and objectively identify some of these factors to the staff. As the nurse's knowledge about cultural factors increases she can identify potential cultural conflict areas, cultural health practices, and cultural norms of the patients, and discuss these factors with the staff. More and more, the nurse will be expected to help educate her health associates about the cultural aspects of patient care, and her teaching methods and techniques should be adapted to the cultural ways in which the staff members can best learn these factors.

Cultural Factors in Patient-Care Situations

Some vignettes of the behavior of patients from different cultural backgrounds will be presented below as illustrative materials to help the reader understand how culture factors can and do influence patient behavior, and to highlight the importance of using cultural background data in giving patient care. These nurse-patient situations are actual ones which the author has observed or encountered.

Situation One: Czech-American Patient. Mrs. S., a 48-year-old Czech-American patient, was admitted to a psychiatric hospital because she was depressed and would not eat. A family informant said that Mrs. S. roamed about the house at night and refused to go to bed. Mrs. S.'s only daughter was too upset to bring her mother to the hospital and so her Anglo-American son-in-law brought her there. The patient spoke only a few sentences in English, but could speak the Czech language well.

The known history of the patient was brief and sketchy. The nurse, however, learned from the son-in-law that the patient came to the United States at the age of 28 years. A year later, her only daughter was born, and Mrs. S. was very happy with the child, Agatha. In a short time, Mrs. S.'s husband died suddenly of a heart attack. This was a great shock to her. Mrs. S. continued to live in this Czech-speaking rural community in northern Ohio. In order to provide for her attractive blonde daughter and herself, she did domestic work in the community, working long hours each day. A few years ago, Mrs. S.'s daughter married to a man whom Mrs. S. did not know very well. The onset of Mrs. S.'s emotional illness began shortly after the marriage. She became depressed, refused to eat, and became easily irritated. Frequently, Mrs. S. would shout at her son-in-law with profane words. The daughter and the son-in-law, who had lived with the mother for one year after their marriage, moved to a separate dwelling nearby. Mrs. S. disliked the fact that her daughter had left her, and soon she made a suicide attempt and became markedly depressed.

Upon admission to the hospital, Mrs. S. was quiet, silently angry, and depressed. She spoke mainly in Czech, but occasionally the nurse could hear her mumbling, "I was always a good mother ... I took care of her ... I cooked good food for her and raised her ... Now she has left me." It was apparent that she was speaking of her daughter. Mrs. S. would pace the hospital corridors and stare at the nursing staff.

The psychiatric team discussed Mrs. S.'s behavior and noted some differences in her behavior when compared with their usual Anglo-American patients in the hospital. They noted that she was "locked up-tight" in talking about her problems. Her mannerisms and thought content were not really typical of a "classical depressed patient." The staff was baffled about the patient's behavior, and were unable to get close to the patient to understand her problems. The author spent time with the patient and obtained considerable psychocultural and social data about the patient and her family. The patient revealed how much she was still living by her traditional Czech cultural norms, rather than by American norms. Mrs. S. talked about how hard she had worked all her life, and especially since her husband's death, in order to provide basic needs for her daughter. She said she was a good mother, since she provided food and clothing for her daughter and had always prepared special foods for her. She was proud of her daughter and loved her very much, until she married an Anglo-American man whom she felt was not warm and friendly to her. When her daughter moved away from her, Mrs. S. became very angry and sad; it was a time of major crisis in her life. She interpreted the daughter's marriage and separation from her as an open and hostile sign of rejection. She thought the daughter and son-in-law had not appreciated the many sacrifices that Mrs. S. had made to raise her daughter under trying circumstances. This history is quite in keeping with Czech cultural norms in that a Czech mother is generally very close to and possessive of her children. She is attentive to them and often gives them special foods and attention. In return, the offspring are expected to be obedient, respectful and deferent to their parents.

While Mrs. S. was in the hospital, she revealed other Czech behavior in that she would provoke reproaches by offering food to patients and then unobtrusively withholding it from them. Her pattern of communicating with the nurses was similar to this food-giving and food-withholding behavior which had manifested itself in her relations with her daughter at an earlier time. Mrs. S. would make positive comments to the nurse and then make a negative statement. This behavior revealed the need of the Czech mother to avoid exaggeration so that a positive statement calls to mind a negative one almost simultaneously. For example, Mrs. S. would say, "My daughter is good, she's terrible, but I know she will make a good mother." During Mrs. S.'s hospitalization, she projected her intense anger about her daughter on the nurses, and her ambivalent feelings about her son-in-law were directed toward the physicians.

A psychiatric nurse clinician spent much time with Mrs. S., assuming largely a daughter role with the patient. She talked with Mrs. S. about her angry feelings toward the daughter and son-in-law in light of culturally defined normative behavior expectations. The nurse helped Mrs. S. to get similar kinds of daughter-mother satisfactions by having other friends come to visit her at home. She helped the patient to become less dependent and emotionally tied to her daughter. The patient's recovery was slow, but favorable. After Mrs. S. was dismissed from the hospital, the nurse visited her each week and helped her to develop interests in her church and community activities. The daughter and son-in-law were also encouraged to visit occasionally with Mrs. S. and not to isolate themselves completely from her.

In this patient study situation, an on-going close nurse-patient relationship was essential in understanding the cultural and emotional ties between the mother and daughter. The nurse helped to move the patient toward new life interests and to reexamine her intense interest in and possession of her daughter. The staff reached the patient only after an understanding of the cultural behavior of Mrs. S. and her family which was obtained with the help of a nurse-anthropologist.

Situation Two: Mexican-American Patient. A Mexican-American mother and her three-year-old daughter were sitting in an outpatient clinic, and soon a nursing student came to them and spoke to them in a warm and friendly manner. This young student was attracted to the child and began to talk positively about the child's beauty and healthy appearance. The nursing student stood about a foot and a half from the mother as she praised the child, but she did not touch her. The broad smile, friendly hand gestures, and favorable comments of the student were all indications that she was warmly admiring the child.

As the student was praising and admiring the child, the mother became noticeably restless about the student's behavior. She began to move restlessly in her chair, and made several attempts to change the position of the child so that the child would not be directly facing the student. The mother's behavior was purposeful. Unknowingly, the nursing student was casting an evil eye (*mal ojo*) on the daughter. The student who was admiring the child was not knowledgeable about the cultural practices and beliefs of the Mexican-American. She had not touched the child, which would have disspelled the force of the evil eye. This behavior on the part of the student was of serious concern to the mother, for the mother knew the consequences of such acts. Interestingly, the student thought that the mother had not understood her kind praises to her daughter, and so she began to reaffirm her verbal and gestural communication by telling the mother openly and directly that her child was "very pretty, strong, and healthy." Consequently, the mother again revealed how extremely uncomfortable she was with the student by putting her belongings in her handbag and getting ready to leave the clinic. About this time, the nursing student was called away from the mother and child. The mother quickly picked up the child and left the clinic.

After the mother and child reached their home, the mother immediately called upon her midwife friends, who are known as *parteras*. She told them what had happened at the clinic and asked that the *parteras* counteract the spell cast on the child by the nursing student. Later, the mother conferred with a native health practitioner called a *curanderos*. He offered her additional advice about the situation. The mother and the indigenous health advisors made the diagnosis that the child was under the influence of malevolent magical forces because of the behavior of the nursing student toward the child. To test this belief, the child's skin was rubbed with substance from a broken egg. A red spot appeared on the child's body, and this confirmed that an evil eye had been cast on her while the student admired her without rubbing her head. The culturally prescribed way to cure the child was to have the person (the student) responsible for causing the evil eye rub the child's head; however, the mother was afraid to return to the clinic and thereby expose the child to more danger. So the mother and her native curers treated the child at home with several treatment methods intended to counteract the malevolent forces of an evil eye.

Situation Three: Afro-American Patient. A 40-year-old Southern black patient was admitted to a hospital in the midwest for an appendectomy. He was placed in a four-bed ward with three Anglo-American patients, and was then taken immediately to surgery. After the surgery the patient went to the recovery room, and later in the day returned to his ward room. After the first post-operative day, Mr. P. appeared fearful, distrustful, and suspicious of the nursing staff, and yet he was dependent upon them for help, food, concern, physical care, and other nursing care measures. Mr. P. revealed that he was suspicious of others by his constant staring at the nurses and by his comments. Frequently, he would say to the men in the ward, "Do you trust those nurses? I don't. I am afraid of what they will do to you and to me. I don't think they really want to help me, but they have to take care of us. I wonder what they will do to me."

The nurses who had not heard these comments from Mr. P. continued to care for him, and did not show any differences between the amount and quality of care they offered to Mr. P. and that which they were offering to the other male patients on the ward. Mr. P. noticed this behavior but kept thinking they would not care for him. One day Mr. P. openly expressed his feelings and concerns to a nurse as she was taking care of his surgical dressing. He spoke rapidly and angrily, saying, "You white folks, I can't trust you completely. You have been taking care of me, but I know you would rather not help me. It has always been that way. It is how I have seen it before and back home." The nurse listened to him and said, "I know you probably doubt if we truly want to help you, but we do. We try to give care to people regardless of their skin color, as we are commited to helping any person in need of nursing care." This comment was spoken in a kind and firm manner which was quite reassuring to Mr. P. It seemed to allay his suspicious behavior, and he was more comfortable with the staff during the remainder of his stay in the hospital.

From a cultural viewpoint, Mr. P.'s suspicious and doubtful behavior might have been anticipated, for he was raised in the South where help and care to black people by the whites is not commonplace. This Southern man is generally in a position where he cannot and does not expect services or help from those who are in a social and economic position superior to his. The behavior of the nurses seemed incongruent to Mr. P. who had expected an inconsistent status situation where there would be differential treatment toward him. It was a questionable and difficult experience to have a white person give him services, when he doubted that any white nurse could be genuinely interested in him. When Mr. P. is at home, he constantly gives personal services to white people; and now, during his hospitalization, the reverse role practices were occurring. How strange it must have seemed to him! This reversal in role behavior occurred so unexpectedly for Mr. P. that he had limited time to adjust to a new behavior after becoming accustomed to one pattern of behavior for nearly forty years. The nurse's comment reassured Mr. P. that she was willing to care for him, and her consistent behavior in giving care to him reaffirmed her verbal comments.

Another interesting cultural feature of the situation was that in Mr. P.'s family structure, men are rather dependent upon females for personal care in the home, and especially in crisis situations. So the female nurse was cast into a cultural role which was helpful to Mr. P. The patient's greatest problem was to be comfortable in accepting care from a white nurse. There was evidence, however, that he was trying to accept the situation and he did in fact accept it toward the end of his hospital stay. The three white nurses working on the ward were born and raised in the northern rural community and had been taught to work with people of different ethnic origins and so they did not experience some of the conflicts that Mr. P. did. They were, on the whole, at ease with Mr. P. and were able to maintain an effective relationship with him.

Situation Four: Swedish-American Patient. Mr. C., a fifty-year-old man of Swedish-American descent (second generation), was admitted to a general hospital with an acute myocardial infarction. He had lived all of his life on a prosperous small farm in central Minnesota in a community populated by other Swedish-American people. His devoted wife and two children had always been active in helping Mr. C. with his 320-acre farm. In recent years, his son and daughter had gotten married and lived in a small town about twenty miles from their parents. Mrs. C. was an active woman who enjoyed community and home activities.

In examining Mr. C.'s Swedish cultural background, we found a number of traditional Swedish features. Mr. C. had been an extremely hard-working man ever since he was a small boy working with his father. He had been a successful farmer and small cattle-raiser. His frugal ways had helped him to get along with what he had, especially during the drought years. He had been an ambitous man, who had provided well for his wife and children. Mr. and Mrs. C. and his family were of the Lutheran faith and regularly attended church services and practiced their beliefs. In the past, Mr. C. enjoyed going fishing at a nearby lake, but lately the pressures of farm life and of having less help from his children had increased his daily farm activities, leaving less time for fishing and other outdoor recreational activities. During the past three years, Mr. C. had felt "driven and pushed" to keep up with his farmwork. He had not relinquished any of his farm land, cattle, and farm activities, for he felt "he could manage all of it." However, he had worried about his ability to deal with the multiple problems arising each day on the farm. Undoubtedly, these concrete pressures were having a definite impact upon Mr. C.'s health state, and could well have been the precipitating factors leading to his heart attack.

Mr. C. did not want to come to the hospital. He wanted to remain at home and have his wife care for him. He said, "I don't want to go to the hospital. Why can't the doctor come to see me at my home?" However, Mr. C.'s acute illness necessitated that he be treated in the hospital. While in the hospital, many Swedish cultural features were evident in his behavior. Mr. C. remained a tight-lipped and quiet man. He seldom talked freely, and volunteered only a few choice words when he felt like talking. When the staff encouraged him to discuss how he felt, he became more tight-lipped than ever. Mr. C.'s pattern of communication also revealed how frightened and tense he was about his illness and what might happen to him. This was his first major illness and the first time he had been in a hospital. Mr. C. remained unusually quiet and noncommunicative to the staff. Most of the time he read and prayed. The staff realized how Mr. C. was feeling and wanted to talk with him, but he was not responsive. Gradually, the nurses discovered that a good way to reach him culturally and psychologically was to offer him a glass of fruit juice and a cookie and then sit silently and have a glass of juice with him. This was a good strategy, as social companionship by the sharing of food is a cultural feature which is enjoyed by Swedish people. They like to have family and friends eat with them, for it provides a natural and casual way to interact with others. Food to the Swedish people is an important medium by which to relate to other people. With this regular "Swedish social break," the nurses reached Mr. C. and began to identify his fears and concerns. They were able to help him relax as they talked casually about his illness and what had happened to him. Gradually, he told them some of his concerns about being in the hospital and whether he could remain on the farm. Although Mr. C. would have preferred a good cup of strong Swedish-brewed coffee, he accepted fruit juices and milk as he related to the nurses and others.

In time, Mr. C. made a good recovery. Another important factor contributing to Mr. C.'s recovery was the daily visit by his wife and children. Mr. C. looked forward to the family members' visit each day. He asked personal questions about them and his farm. He was worried about the farm and whether anyone was taking good care of it. He was reassured by his children that an old farm friend had come to take care of the place for him. As might be culturally expected, Mr. C.'s wife and daughter always brought a sack full of home-made cookies and other Swedish goodies to Mr. C. when they came to see him. Mr. C.'s eyes and hands indicated that this—plus their coming to see him—was the best gift ever. He shared the cookies with other patients and the nursing staff during their morning, afternoon, and evening "Swedish social breaks." The cookies were cultural symbols of family love and social interest which linked Mr. C. close to his friends, home, family, and community. Mr. C.'s recovery was slow, but he was able to go home after two months of hospitalization. Gradually, he was able to let others farm his land and take care of the heavy farm chores. He was able to return to the farm and live as if he were a city-farmer doing only minor farm activities.

Situation Five: Cheyenne Indian and Anglo-American Couple. A 23-year-old Cheyenne Indian husband and his 25-year-old Anglo-American wife had been referred to a neighborhood mental health clinic to receive marital counseling. It was the wife's Anglo neighbors who had urged them to come to the clinic for help. The husband was hesitant to come.

Mr. and Mrs. D. had been married for three years, but were unhappy after the first child was born (one year after their marriage). Mr. D.'s chief complaint was that his wife was "too noisy and talkative, and was not a good mother, as she was constantly yelling at their two children and physically punishing them severely with a strap or stick." The Anglo-American wife (middle-lower class) was angry with her husband because he was "too quiet, passive, and did not discipline their two children enough." She also complained that her Indian husband was always embarrassed when he talked to her Anglo-American friends. This bothered Mrs. D. considerably because her Anglo friends complained to her about her husband's inability to look at and talk to them.

At the mental health clinic, the wife candidly talked about a number of her husband's annoying behavior traits, and she was quick to elaborate her points with many detailed examples. In contrast, the husband appeared embarrassed about his wife talking so blatantly about him, and said very little about her. Mr. D. seemed to take the criticism as if it was his duty or obligation. The wife complained particularly and bitterly that her husband never physically disciplined the children. She said, "They will be so spoiled when they get big ... If you spare the rod, you'll spoil the child ... I had lots of punishment when I was growing up and punishment is good for children. They need it." The husband shook his head and stared at her, but would not talk about the problems of disciplining the children.

The contrastive behaviors of Mr. and Mrs. D. were understandable from a cultural viewpoint. Let us consider the Cheyenne Indians' way of living, and we will soon realize that this man and woman were raised in two entirely different worlds. This was the crux of their marital difficulties. The Cheyenne Indians, who call themselves "The People," are one of the most respected and interesting Indian groups of the Great Plains. Hoebel states, "Their attitudes toward sex and war, and toward the maintenance of their social order, are the outstanding features of their way of life."[1] The Cheyenne Indians are famous for the courage of their warriors, and the bravery and chastity of their women. In their early culture history, they were outstanding warriors, effective gardeners, and nomadic hunters. However, their way of life has changed through the years, and today they are living in cities and trying to adjust to an industrial way of life.

The adult personality of the Cheyenne male is reserved and dignified. He moves with a quiet sense of self-respect and self-assurance. He speaks, but never in a wasteful or careless manner, for he is kind and generous to the feelings of others. Generally he is slow to get angry, and seldom does he become openly aggressive unless continually aggravated. During the course of Cheyenne socialization practices, he was taught to suppress his feelings, especially toward kinsmen, affines, and friends. However, toward enemies he feels no merciful compunctions, and he can become very aggressive in battle-like situations. The Cheyenne people are known to have a firm grip on reality and to deal with problems in well-defined ways, and yet they are capable of adjusting to new situations if the reasons seem logical and realistic. As the Cheyenne man matures, he is serene, composed and capable of warm social relations. Certainly he has anxieties, but he usually knows how to control them appropriately by means of self-discipline. According to our cultural norms, the Cheyenne are shy and reserved people, and it has been said that they are given to feelings of shame in direct social intercourse and especially in contact with strangers. They seldom look directly at people, but rather gaze at the ground or at a point some distance away from the person who is speaking. The Cheyenne wife and mother exhibits much the same behavior, except that she is probably more creative than the male in handling aggressive tendencies, since she has only minimal approved outlets for aggression.

As one examines briefly the child-rearing practices of the Cheyenne child, one becomes impressed with the high value placed upon children. From birth, the child is loved, wanted, and cared for tenderly. Ideally, the child grows in an atmosphere of love and interest. He is rarely physically punished. Crying babies are not scolded nor physically abused. Instead, they are taken from their cradleboards and given love. Occasionally, parents let the child cry to help him realize that loss of social contact is non-rewarding. But in general, the infants and children are cuddled, constantly loved, and rocked in the arms of their mother and maternal kinsmen. Children at a young age are taught to be quiet and respectful, mainly by imitation of their parents' subtle mannerisms and covert love. Love and respect move the child to want to emulate adults and engage in adult activities. A soft voice and persuasive verbal comments are used when dealing with children. Furthermore, the Cheyenne mother is submissive to her husband and takes cues from him in ways to handle a child.

The Cheyenne cultural ways are a drastic contrast with those of Mrs. D., a middle-lower class Anglo-American woman; in fact, the cultural norms seem almost the opposite. Mrs. D. was raised to be assertive, aggressive, disrespectful, and outspoken to her husband. She had been reared by punitive parents who frequently punished her physically if she did not obey them. Physical punishment was the believed-in and desired norm for controlling children and making them into good adults. Mrs. D. had received many "beltings" and abuses from her parents. She was taught that the only way a child can be made to understand what you wanted him to do was by talking loudly and firmly to him, and then by using physical punishment to reinforce the "lecture." The women from her culture were aggressive and were taught not to be deferent to males.

Although one could continue to identify other contrastive features between the two cultures, these were the crucial points to show that the cultural backgrounds of Mr. and Mrs. D. were noticeably different and were the major factors in causing marital stress. Differences in child-rearing techniques, parental attitudes, and role behavior of a husband and wife were sources which caused marital tensions. Most significant, however, were the markedly different attitudes of each spouse regarding ways to rear a child. As described above, the child-rearing norms were almost the opposite in the two cultures. How could a husband and wife resolve such difficulties?

The couple had come for help, and so the psychiatric team proceeded to analyze their marital problems. It soon became apparent that cultural differences were so great that an anthropologist was sought to give consultation to the team. Accordingly, the above data were highlighted by the anthropologist and special treatment plans were formulated based upon this information. The therapy continued largely by helping the couple realize the differences in their cultural backgrounds and what compromises and adjustments they wanted to make about these differences. They struggled with the problems, but it was extremely difficult for either of them to yield to another way of living.

With the recent practice of intercultural marriages, this patient study situation is becoming more common. As nurses, we need to be cognizant of such cultural differences and how they influence marriage relationships. It would have been impossible to work with this couple if the anthropologist had not been brought into the situation to help the staff understand the crux of the problem. The psychiatric team was open and willing to have an anthropologist participate in its group sessions. In this chapter, only a few nurse-patient study examples have been given to disclose the ways cultural factors influence patient behavior. Needless to say, many other examples can be found today in health settings.

FOOTNOTES

[1] E. Adamson Hoebel, *The Cheyennes: Indians of the Great Plains*, New York: Holt, Rinehart and Winston, Inc., 1960, p. 1.

8 The Cultural Context of Behavior: Spanish-Americans and Nursing Care

In this chapter the cultural context of human behavior will be examined with respect to one particular cultural group, namely, the Spanish-Americans. An understanding of the cultural context of human behavior is important to health personnel for gaining an in-depth view of the people one is working with and to help one discover ways to tailor-make treatment and nursing care plans.[1] The cultural context approach strives for *specificity* in the consideration of patient problems and for *reducing ambiguity in nursing goals*. The approach gives full support to the discovery of cultural factors influencing or determining an individual or group health problem.

Meaning of the Cultural Context of Behavior

The cultural context of behavior refers to the implicit and explicit behavior tendencies of a designated group of people who have lived and interacted together in a particular cultural setting according to certain values, practices, and life goals. Each cultural group in various places in the world has its own life style, its own patterns of living, and its own special way of viewing the world about it. Its special world view is the essential basis of a people's modes of acting and thinking, and its world view serves as the basic framework for their unique cultural context of behavior. The cultural context of behavior is, however, shaped and maintained by social, politicalm religious, economical, kinship, historical, and specific cultural factors. These factors are interdigitated and produce a certain pattern of behavior which gives "Character" and distinction to a culture's mode of living. As one studies the cultural context of behavior, it is important to see how these various elements fit together to provide a comprehensive picture of the people. The behavior of certain individuals or sub-groups makes sense when perceived within the cultural context of behavior, one can predict the behavior tendencies with a fair degree of accuracy.

Anthropologists believe that one of the best ways to understand the meaning and significance of the cultural context of behavior is to become active participants in the life ways of a particular culture. Perhaps one might choose to live with a group of people for a period of time in order to gain special knowledge about the ways they interact with each other. A conscious effort must be made to know a particular group's way of living, and this effort must be directed largely towards *seeing and hearing through the eyes and ears of the people.* Empathy, interest, objectivity, and involvement are crucial means of grasping the cultural context behavior. A study of the daily, weekly, monthly, and yearly life activities of people blended with social science data about a given group can insure a good overview of the contextual aspects of human behavior. It is rewarding to put bits and pieces of cultural data together so that a larger and meaningful picture comes into existence. The whole process of determining the cultural context of behavior is analogous to putting a jig-saw puzzle together. Generally, the pieces will fit together if one is willing to struggle with the idea of a gestalt view. Since nurses may find it difficult to live with a cultural group (although it is highly recommended by this author), an alternative approach to grasping the cultural context of behavior is to be an active listener, observer, and good questioner about the people one desires to know. In addition, one can draw upon the knowledge in the literature to know "one's people." With this in mind, we turn to an exploration of the cultural context features of the Spanish-American peoples as an example of how to go about understanding the many-faceted dimensions of a cultural group.

The Cultural Context of the Spanish-American

General Cultural Features. The Spanish-American people are descendants of the Spanish colonists, who date back to the eighteenth century.[2] It is generally agreed that the exact location of the Spanish colonization and cultural heritage in the United States includes the present New Mexico, Arizona, Texas, southern and central California, southern Colorado, and the east coast of Florida. Many of these Spanish-Americans share distinctive cultural features which influence their behavior in spite of their continuous contacts with other cultural groups in our society.

At the outset, it is important to clarify that the Spanish-Americans, Mexican-Americans, and Mexicans are three major subgroups of the total Spanish-speaking population. Each of these subgroups has its own cultural ways and beliefs and historical background, and so one cannot view them as identical in cultural behavior. Through time, however, there have been various kinds of interaction with a wide variety of other cultural and subcultural groups in the United States, which have shaped certain aspects of their behavior to make them similar in certain respects with one another.

The Spanish-Americans are the remaining descendants of the old Spanish colonial group who came into the middle and upper Rio Grande valleys. These people are referred to as "hispanos," and their largest populations are concentrated in New Mexico and southern Colorado. When the Spanish colonists came to America, a low ratio of women to men existed among them, and so wives were sought among the indigenous Indian populations of the region. Intermarriage with the American Indians was a common practice until the early nineteenth century; and, marriage between the Anglo-Americans the Spanish increased. The Spanish-American of today is a genetic descendant of sixteenth and seventeenth century Spain, and of the new Spain with some intermarriage with the American Indians and with Anglo-Americans.

The Spanish-Americans tend to hold themselves aloof from the Mexican-Americans, since they recognize their past heritage ties while of course, Mexican-Americans cherish their own rich background. Through the years, however, Mexican-Americans and Spanish-Americans have shown some cultural similarities because of their intermarriage practices and their ways of dealing with common social, political, and economic problems. From the Mexican-American's physical appearance, one can see a closer tie with the Indian culture of America than with the Spanish-Americans. Physical characteristics, however, are but a small aspect of the total factors influencing any culture's behavior and way of living.

Spanish-Americans became citizens of the United States by military conquest which involved no immediate necessity to modify their traditional way of life, no substantive break with their cultural traditions, and no change in residence. Today there are about 500,000 Spanish-Americans in rural and urban areas of the southwest United States.

Social and Kinship Aspects. The social life of the Spanish-American was traditionally organized (as it still is largely today) around the extended family and the church. The father is the patriarch whose authority is recognized and expected to be exercised. He is responsible for giving guidance and leadership to the family, and for making all major decisions. The role of the mother and wife is subordinate to her husband or to the father of the household. The mother's interests are primarily in bearing children, and in caring for her family, her home, and her close kinsmen. The father and husband is expected to assume material responsibility for his wife and children. His private or personal morals are his own business, but his social or group morals must be above reproach if he is to maintain his status in the family and the community. The eldest son has authority over younger siblings and has a right to influence the mother regarding family decisions. The extended and nuclear family in the rural and urban areas binds the Spanish-American family together, so that family matters always prevail over individual and non-family affairs.

Kinship ties extend beyond the biological ties within the family to the important institution known as *compadrasgo*, or godparents, who maintain a strong religious and social obligation toward the child. Grandparents are highly respected for their decisions and are frequently consulted for their opinions about family problems. All family and kin members are expected to show respect for one another.

The family is the chief link with the community and provides a model for relationships outside the kinship group. The family members have definite steps they follow regarding who treats illness and what specific role each person should play. The mother is first to become aware of the child or adult's illness, and then the mother seeks the father's advice. Next they seek the mother's mother for advice, and then the godparents or co-parents (*compadres*). If the family remedies do not prove efficious, then the indigenous lay medical people are sought, namely, the *medicas, sobadors, curanderos,* and *albolarios*. Finally, professional or non-indigenous practitioners may be sought, particularly if the individual is seriously ill and death seems imminent. Thus the family is the group of unity and the group which deals first with a health problem. This is one of the major reasons why many physicians, nurses, and others have wondered why Spanish-American people are slow to come for professional help. Professional health personnel must realize that these people have their own health care and treatment system, including their own practitioners with whom they feel most comfortable and secure. Many Spanish-Americans still tend to seek non-indigenous help only when an illness is extremely serious or threatening to the life of a family member. There are, of course, some Spanish-Americans who are highly acculturated to Anglo-American middle and middle-upper class practices, and they seek professional help at an early time.

Religious Aspects. The Spanish-Americans are predominantly of the Roman Catholic faith. A small percent are Protestant or have another religious affiliation. Traditionally, religion was a significant factor in the people's lives, for it helped to unify and integrate their total life ways in the family and in the community. In recent years, religion has not been such a powerful force in the lives of the Spanish-American people. There is less ritualism and fewer daily religious activities; moreover, some of the major feasts and ceremonies of the Church are celebrated with less elaboration and fewer signs of external pious devotion. Nevertheless, varying degrees of religious faith continue to serve important functions and purposes for these people. It is common to hear some Spanish-Americans express regret that the ceremonial and religious activities of the Catholic Church are waning and changing. The priest continues to be recognized in many Spanish-American communities as the people's spiritual leader, and he serves as a counselor regarding temporal, religious, and community matters.

Political Aspects. Politics and political strivings are well known to the Spanish-American people, and are more apparent in some parts of their territory than others. For example, in the State of New Mexico political action has been quite noticeable in furthering the people's desires for land and general national rights. The Spanish-Americans in this state comprise more than one-half the total population of the state, and they are actively using political processes to control and protect their rights. In other states where Spanish-Americans reside, political action is not as forceful as it was in the past; however, there are today more apparent signs of overt political activity. It can be anticipated that as Spanish-Americans become more involved in national and state affairs, their traditional political methods will change along with the problems they seek to resolve. Contrary to the general public image, the Spanish-American people are not as passive and non-aggressive people as one might think them to be. When their rights, privileges and goals are at stake, they are willing to fight for them. They have been known through their culture history to rise actively and firmly to deal with matters affecting their well being.

Political leadership emanates from the male leader of the household who learns to become a good speaker and defender of the family and community. Currently, Spanish-Americans are becoming active in Anglo-American politics in order to share in our nation's wealth, to establish democratic freedom and protection, and to obtain material, social, and political rights in our American society. New young political leaders are emerging among the Spanish-Americans, who have learned through our educational system and life experience how to obtain American rights. Reies Lopez Tijerina, for example, has been extremely active in strengthening the political movement for return of grant land to Southwest Hispanos.[3] Spanish-Americans are fighting politically for better living facilities, good schools, adequate food, and other kinds of public assistance. Political behavior as a way of influencing others to gain self and group help has changed through the years for the Spanish-American peoples, and now their behavior is becoming similar to that of many Anglo-Americans. And it is reasonable to predict that the Spanish-Americans will continue to be more open and active in national affairs than they have been in the past.

Economic Aspects. The Spanish-American way of community life has traditionally been based upon agriculture. In the past, the small irrigated farm was a prosperous and self-sufficient means of supporting a family. Today, those who have retained their lands are finding it difficult to support their large families because of rising costs related to modern technological and general farming expenses. Those who have no land live as tenants, sharecroppers, or are hired by farmers who own land. Many have joined the streams of migrant agricultural laborers who travel here and there seeking employment on sugar beet, potato, fruit, or small grain farms. As migrant farmers they find it difficult to improve their economic status, and often they go for years without any improvement in their economic status. There is, however, considerable value, among Spanish-Americans, placed on possessing their own land and raising their own crops for their family and friends. Most of the land they own is semi-arid, with limited irrigation systems. Modern irrigation and farm machinery are rarely found on their acreages. Cattle and sheep-raising supplements their livelihood. Cattle, sheep and goats are often a major source of their income, along with products from their gardens.

Industries in and near the cities have attracted many Spanish-Americans to work as unskilled and semi-skilled laborers. Only a few years ago, agriculture was the mainstay of their economy, with family wage work to supplement their agricultural production. Today, wage and salary work is the principal means of a Spanish-American's livelihood. Many families now engage in agricultural activities primarily to provide fresh food for family use and to keep "in touch" with their past cultural interests.

Only a small proportion of Spanish-Americans are wealthy. In general, their living facilities are modest and their economic status is meager (whether they live in rural or urban areas). Most Spanish-Americans have had approximately eight years or less of formal education so that it is difficult for them to compete in the industrial world with Anglo-Americans and others. Then, too, many of the Spanish-Americans speak the Spanish language and have difficulty in speaking English fluently, and this often limits what jobs are available to them. Urbanization trends continue to bring the Spanish-American people into the cities, where educational facilities are more accessible to them. There is some concern and hesitation, however, about sending Spanish-American children to these Anglo-oriented schools because parents fear the consequences of the schools' emphasis on competition, open aggression and high achievement—all values contrary to the traditional Spanish-American way of life. Then, too, they feel the children should work at home or along with their parents in their unskilled jobs in order to maintain a continuity of livelihood in the urban community.

Class differences among the Spanish-Americans do exist and range from the lower class, who are often isolated farm villagers, to a small core of upper class people who enjoy the status of their old family traditions and family wealth or who have achieved wealth in our modern society. Those who are fully acculturated to the modern American life may have today's technological conveniences and live as middle class citizens. Interestingly enough, some Spanish-Americans who have been exposed to modern ways have not given up their older life style. Doubts and suspicions exist among some Spanish-Americans about Anglo-American values and practices which they fear might change drastically or weaken their family and group life.

Health-Illness Systems. In the course of time, the Spanish-Americans have used a variety of sources for their knowledge about diseases and the treatment of illness. They have drawn upon: (1) the folk medical lore of medieval Spain; (2) the health-illness treatment practices of American Indians, especially the Mexican Indians; and (3) the Anglo folk and modern medical practices found in rural and urban areas. These sources of knowledge have deen combined with their own health-illness system and adapted to other aspects of their culture.

Traditionally, the Spanish-American health-illness system was closely interwoven with faith and fatalism, and any illness could be explained; this system prepared people psychologically and culturally for life uncertainties. Their strong faith in God and their kinsmen helped to sustain them in accepting a disease and in maintaining their beliefs. Their philosophy and values of human life also helped them realize that not all of life can be fully controlled by man. To them, normal health was always subject to attack and change, just as sin and temptation always existed in the world. There was no such thing as perfect health, for health is relative to an individual and his situation. Spanish-American people realize that illness exists because perfection in health never exists completely. Being able to function adequately means wellness even though such adequacy may involve the actual malfunctioning of a body part. Good and evil are always present and are conflicting forces in man's life; so one meets and accepts illness and death, sadness and joy, good and evil.

Man is faced with the challenge of keeping his body in a state of balance or equilibrium in order to be healthy. Since the body is seen as a functioning whole, operations are viewed as dangerous to bodily wholeness. Man's body must function as a whole with the maintenance of a balance of hot and cold substances in the body. For example: (1) If your feet get wet, it is important to get your head wet, since an imbalance will lead to a sore throat; (2) One should use chili (hot food) to treat pneumonia (cold disease); (3) Avoid citrus fruits (cold food) as they will cause colic; (4) Drinking cold water after a hot day may cause *empacho* (indigestion). Balance must also be maintained in emotional expressions and interpersonal relationships.

Many Spanish-American people believe that they have limited control over nature. They believe that God gives health and that he sends illness to them for some reason. They recognize that some diseases are caused by accidents, the devil, witchcraft, heredity, and so on. However, they say that ultimately all diseases are caused by God. God is seen as merciful in that he gives knowledge to medical people so they can be physicians, *medicas*, or *medicos*, and can help people. An unbending faith in God and a faith in curing are essential to recovery; moreover, the cure or lack of cure is in God's hands, not in the hands of human beings. Although Spanish-Americans are knowledgeable about preventive measures and their importance, they do not necessarily think that preventive remedies are of primary relevance if an individual suddenly becomes ill, because God may have willed the illness.

A misfortune such as illness can be viewed either as a punishment from God (*castigo de Dios*) or as a cross to bear. Mental illness and mental retardation are crosses to bear for the family members. So God is primarily in charge of health, and can cause or permit illness. Pregnancy is viewed as normal, and so health personnel should not disrupt something which God controls. Accordingly, a child is in the hands of God, and it is hard to understand why immunizations are considered so important and extoiled so hard by health workers. This acceptance of and resignation to God's will provides emotional comfort and explanations of illness and health, and prepares Spanish-American people for many unexpected daily happenings and misfortunes which man faces everywhere. An assault from the unknown (*prendido*), a mysterious power influencing others, and general misfortunes can be accepted if one believes that supernatural forces control man and nature.[4]

To the Spanish-American, a healthy person is one who looks and acts healthy. A healthy adult is well proportioned, has good color, good muscles, and does a good day's work. A healthy child is plump and rosy; he eats well and is physically active. A sick person is unable to do daily routine activities and has lost strength and weight. Health is essentially a day-to-day state of being which is governed by natural and supernatural forces shaping the present. A person has to feel discomfort, otherwise he is not ill. There is limited emphasis upon causes of illness, since Spanish-American people know what probably caused the illness—either an evil force or God's will.

Diseases are classified primarily as physical or natural diseases. Some of these are similar to diseases found among Mexican-American peoples.[5] Four of the common indigenous diseases are the following:

1. *Mal ojo*, literally translated "bad eye," is a disease which is believed to afflict a person (usually a child) because someone admires or desires the child to an excessive degree. The afflicted person becomes

ill with symptoms of sleepiness, general malaise, and excessive tiredness. The treatment is to find the person who has cast the "evil eye" and have him (her) caress or touch the person. Prophylactically, when a person admires a child, he should always touch the child. This gestures reduces the spell being cast on the child and protects him from illness.

2. *Empacho* is a condition in which food forms into a ball and clings to the wall of the stomach, preventing the assimilation of food. Generally, the cause of *empacho* is the poor quality of food given to an individual because of a malicious contamination of the food by a personal enemy. Stomach cramps and nervousness are common symptoms. Treatment includes a combined physical magico-religious practice in which prayers are recited while the spine is massaged gently with small doses of mercury derivative (*greta*). Other treatment modalities are also employed.

3. *Mal de susto*, or "illness from fright," is believed to be the result of an emotionally traumatic experience. The patient becomes frightened, tense, and drowsy, and experiences a loss of energy. Occasionally night sweats are noted. The treatment is directed toward relaxing the individual with herb tea (*llerba buena*) and ritually "sweeping" the person with a branch. Again, prayers are recited during the sweeping ritual. *Susto* is caused by natural fright, such as being nearly injured. In constrast, *espanto* (fright) is caused by seeing a devil or ghost. Sometimes acculturated individuals do not distinguish between these two fright syndromes.

4. *Maleficio*, or witchcraft, is largely caused by witches or malicious friends. It is greatly feared by the people and many preventive steps are taken to avoid being bewitched. Witches are believed to obtain their power from the devil. Often those who are arousing envy and jealousy in others fear that a witch will be used to harm them. Witches can transform themselves into other persons or into animals. Their evil is worked by sympathetic image magic. Some witches force an evil wind (*mal aire*) which can produce acute pain to enter a person's body. In general, witchcraft is greatly feared by the people. They are reluctant to discuss the subject except with close kinsmen, friends, or family members.

Today many familiar diseases are recognized among the Spanish-Americans such as arthritis, asthma, cancer, colds, diarrhea, heart diseases, pneumonia, tuberculosis, etc., but the people frequently recognize different causes and treatments of these diseases than those found acceptable among Anglo-American professionals. Moreover, the Spanish-American people have many remedies for disease states and known health stressors. Herbs are used frequently for ingestion, poultices, infusions, and topical cures. Massage and manipulation for illness are other therapeutic techniques frequently used, and these are referred to as *sobando* and *traqueando*.

Folk practitioners with a variety of skills are used in the treatment of their culturally defined illnesses. These practitioners are still recognized today, and are sought after for their skill in diagnosing and treating an illness. The following practitioners are found in the Spanish-American health-treatment system:[6]

1. A *sobador* is a specialist in massage, who is also known for his ability to handle fractures and bone disorders.
2. A *partera*, or midwife, is usually an older woman who has become an expert in assisting with the delivery of babies. Through the accumulated practical experience of the *parteras* with mothers and infants, she is responsible for the delivery of the infant and provides therapeutic emotional support to the mother. A *partera* has extensive knowledge of folk medicines, especially herbs and the various traditional treatments. In recent years, *parteras* are being recognized by health departments and professional personnel. They are also being exposed to professional views and practices related to maternal and child health care. The synthesis of indigenous and professional health practices should make them a special kind of health worker.
3. A *medico* is a woman or man considered as a general specialist in folk medicine. The *medico* is able to treat a wide variety of illnesses with specific local remedies and/or with therapeutic massage. The *medico* is usually called when a sick person has not responded to general home remedies, or if the family is dissatisfied with modern professional services.
4. A *curandero* is a female and sometimes a male specialist who is equivalent to the Anglo general practitioner. Some *curanderos* are noted specialists for many kinds of diseases. They have a power to heal which they believe is a gift (*don*) from God, and so all treatments are accompanied by propiation to God or one of the saints. Often, *curanderos* have an altar in their consulting rooms. The *curandero* and patient often pray together, and the patient's payment is ritualized to show his awareness that the curer has served as God's means of helping the patient; Generally, the patient leaves an offering before one of the saints. *Curanderos* claim they are inspired by God to become curers. Their training is under other practicing curers or in centers of folk curing. Treatment by a *curandero* is meaningful in the

context of the patient's culture. Generally the family obtains the services of a *curandero* for their ill family member and the family is kept informed of the reasoning behind the diagnosis and the progress of the patient under treatment.
5. ·An *albolario* is a man, or sometimes a woman, who specializes in the treatment of victims of witchcraft. Only a few of these practitioners exist today. Sometimes a man may be known as both a *curandero* and *albolario*. They deal with witches or *brujas*.

It is of interest that when Spanish-Americans go to an Anglo-American practitioner after they have experienced no success with their home remedies, they look for a chiropractor or an osteopath because they manipulate the bones and muscles, a role similar to that of the familiar folk practitioners. In rural areas, folk medicine and folk practitioners are preferred, because of their knowledge of local medicines and the techniques of folk healing. These practitioners also take a high degree of personal interest in the patient, his family, and kinsmen, and the family can participate actively and knowingly in the treatment. Although the state and local health departments in Colorado, New Mexico, and in other states have made noticeable efforts to bring medical and general health services to Spanish-Americans, there are still rural areas which have no modern medical facilities and local folk medical treatment is used.[7] Taos County in New Mexico and Costilla County in Colorado have been places where health services and medical care programs have been established. These programs have not been too successful because they failed to accommodate cultural factors related to the health maintenance and the treatment of disease.[8] Other studies have also stressed the importance of understanding the Spanish-American culture to establish good relationships with the people and to communicate effectively with them if one hopes to have a successful health program.[9,10]

To the Spanish-American, health and illness are largely viewed as existing only in the present time, and there is little emphasis upon illness in the future. The present moment is the major concern to the people and determines how the people respond to questions about health and illness. The comment "*bueno sano*" (or well and hale) means the person is functioning well for the present.

Implications for Nursing

It is obvious that there are differences between Spanish-American and Anglo-American views of the causes, nature, and treatment of diseases; differences exist in their cultural values, beliefs, and practices. The cultural context in which health is maintained, or in which illness develops is a broad and complex framework closely related to political, religious, social, economic, and cultural practices. For Spanish-Americans, health and illness must be assessed and treated with respect to these many factors in the patient's cultural setting. There is a particularly close relationship with the patient's illness and his religious practices and family relationships. The nurse must view wellness and illness of Spanish-Americans in connection with these variables and others, and not see illness as an isolated physical or psychological phenomenon.

In working with a Spanish-American patient and his family, the nurse will be able to understand the full nature of the patient's illness if she can speak or understand the Spanish language. Although many Spanish-Americans are becoming bilingual who live in the United States and especially in urban areas, still there are many persons who cannot speak English. These persons when ill tend to avoid contact with Anglos and to show signs of social isolation. In order to reach these people and understand their health problems, one must understand the language they speak.

Some Anglo-Americans tend to show annoyance to Hispanos who do not know how to speak English and this only aggravates and complicates the nurse reaching the patient's feelings and concerns.[11] When language annoyance occurs between Anglos and Spanish-Americans, there is often the expectation that Spanish-Americans should speak English, not that Anglo-Americans should know Spanish. This behavior implies that members of a subculture should meet the expectations of the dominant culture. As a consequence of such interpersonal encounters and attitudes, poor cooperation and feelings of resentment exist between persons from the two cultures.

Frequently one hears a comment that Spanish-Americans are "lazy," "apathetic" and "irresponsible" people. Again, labeling of a cultural group does not really help to understand the people for it does not convey an accurate picture of the people's behavior. It is a superficial label without clarification of meaning or use. Generally, the "apathetic" and so-called "irresponsible attitude" occurs as a dynamic consequence of the Spanish-American's interaction with an Anglo-American stranger. In the interactional process, the Spanish-American patient is sensitive to the behavior of the Anglo-American and often responds in an initial helpless-like manner as he feels he cannot handle the dominant and often aggressive, perceived attitude of the stranger. He then withdraws socially and appears apathetic. If one understands Spanish-American culture and the many feelings and specific attitude toward strangers, one can see that cultural labeling is superficial with the meaning of behavior being lost in labeling persons.

Gaps and distortions in communication can occur readily as a result of our use of professional expressions as well as through our many nonverbal forms of communication. Since Spanish-Americans are generally polite, deferent, and quiet in an initial encounter with strangers, they often agree with strangers in order to please them. They too may not understand the stranger's behavior and message. Since community health nurses often have contact with these Spanish-American patients in their homes, they can serve as important persons in helping them. They should be patient and allow time to listen to them and try to understand their health problems from their perspective. Most important, nurses should provide explanations which take into account the extent to which the patient and his family are acculturated and they should not assume that all Spanish-American people are equally acculturated. In general, technical and professional terms should be simply defined and clarified. Whenever possible, visual aids should be used to demonstrate health practices. A conscious effort should be made to assess ideas communicated between the patient and the nurse. Still another important communication principle is to look directly at the patient when talking to him, then to listen attentively to his comments and responses and check for the meaning of the message. In the author's recent study of several Spanish-American families, she noted that the people dislike Anglo-Americans talking to them in a hurried manner and maintaining little eye contact while talking to them, as this behavior was interpreted by them as a superficial interest in them as people.

Another way to gain cooperation and establish rapport with Spanish-American people is to use proper forms of address, e.g., saying "Mr. Martinez" rather than using his first name, "Joseph." The nurse, too, should remember to view health problems as private information and to avoid publicizing them. Maintaining an attitude of privacy is important for many reasons, but primarily because Spanish-Americans see illness as a malevolent force with secretive religious and social implications.

Health personnel must realize that it is rather useless to argue persistently with Spanish-Americans in an effort to change their traditional health practices. Instead, if a nurse strives for a warm, friendly, and understanding relationship with the family and remains consciously respectful of their traditional beliefs, she will be more likely to change some of their health practices than if she argues with them. Spanish-Americans accept suggestions and advice about new health practices once a trusting relationship has been established. Spanish-Americans like to view health workers as friends, rather than formal, indifferent, and cold strangers. If the nurse gets to know the Spanish-American family and shows signs of genuine respect and empathy for them, they will be apt to cooperate with her. One can say that the most important professional skill that Spanish-Americans look for in a nurse is her interpersonal skill and her genuine interest in them as a cultural group. This significant professional attribute is possible only when health personnel understand the dynamic cultural context of human behavior and specific cultural groups.

Hanson and Saunders have suggested that professional personnel use the "linkage" concept to help indigenous people.[12] The linkage concept refers to the conscious effort to link the traditional and current beliefs and practices of a cultural group with professional ideas that fit with the indigenous people's health-illness system. The idea of linking the health practices of two cultural groups together is a relevant one, but necessitates that one must understand the differences and similarities between the beliefs and practices of the indigenous and the professional groups. Blending indigenous beliefs and practices with our professional beliefs also requires that professional persons function as highly imaginative and knowledgeable persons about the Spanish-American culture. With the linkage approach, the therapeutic effects and their ties with other social and cultural factors are given consideration. A give-and-take attitude between the nurse and the cultural group she is working with is essential for effective work with people.

Rather than alienating them from the health plans, the professional nurse must consider the important role of the indigenous health practitioners and how they can be utilized in the care and treatment of the patient. Native practitioners are viewed as important persons in the care and treatment of Spanish-American people. They are the practitioners whom the family members call upon first when a serious illness arises, and they are valued for their ideas on ways to prevent illnesses. These practitioners should be perceived by health personnel as an integral part of the people's health-illness system and one should work closely with these people. The belief that all Spanish-Americans are persons who have some role to play in maintaining health or in helping sick persons regain their health state is an important concept to be kept in mind by professional workers. For example, a *medica* must fulfill the role of a confidant to her patients and must maintain a close personal relationship with them. *Medicas* share in the on-going joys of the family as well as in their frustrations and sorrows. They are also important psychotherapists, physical therapists as well as social therapists. To Spanish-Americans, a nurse or physician who shows an impersonal attitude, uses sophisticated language, and gives orders in a formal directive manner, does not fit well with the people's expectations of a good *medicas*. The *medicas* is the people's closest role model for conceptualizing a professional health practitioner. Excessive emotionalism, however, and too personalized behavior with Spanish-American may also create doubts in their minds about one's motives. A nurse who communicates genuine respect, and who offers warmth, friendliness, and overt signs of helpfulness, will be successful in interactions with Spanish-American people.

A full acknowledgement by the nurse of the Spanish-American value orientations is extremely important, and these can be briefly highlighted as follows: (1) man's nature is basically bad, and so normal health is always subject to attack; (2) man must keep his body and mind in a state of balance to be healthy; (3) man has limited control over nature and God; (4) God gives health and sends illness; (5) the present is all-important; (6) the family is the important link between the individual and the outside world; and (7) personalism and being oneself are important to man, especially in his relationship to other men. These cultural values can offer the nurse many important clues for building and maintaining a successful relationship with Spanish-American patients.

In this next section, some relevant nursing care guidelines and suggestions will be summarized. First, in planning and implementing health services for Spanish-American patients, the nurse should give full consideration to the role of the nuclear and extended family. The family is important at every phase of the curing and rehabilitation process. It is highly recommended that the nurse work toward the goal of getting family decisions about health care and treatment rather than relying upon professional pre-made decisions. In addition, individual decisions are not as effective as family group decisions unless the family is highly acculturated to middle class Anglo-American norms. Illness tends to be a social, family, and community matter rather than an illness state of one person.

Second, advice and suggestions will generally be more helpful to the patient and his family than firm directives or "physician-nurse orders." The nurse may need to offer some professional health suggestions, and she does this best by providing clear explanations and some evidence that her health practices have some positive consequences. Findings from specific research studies which are presented in a simple visual and candid manner are often helpful in helping Spanish-Americans understand professional health practices.

Third, if the nurse is working in a Spanish-American community she should involve local health leaders and indigenous health practitioners whenever she can in the health care or program plans. These health workers are generally well known and close to the Spanish-American people who take pride in seeing that local people are active participants in health activities. Health programs conducted by strangers to the community are seldom as effective as they are when the local people have an active part in the program. Of course, this is an important principle for successful work with any cultural or social group.

Fourth, ritual acts are important to Spanish-Americans. The nurse should be familiar with the positive values of ritualized health practices and ways to use rituals in helping people remain healthy. Ritual health practices can be used in the care of infants, in planning diets, and in teaching techniques for preventing the spread of contagious diseases or other illnesses. In bathing an infant, using each the same techniques, equipment, and sequence of activities would help establish a ritual health practice. Ritual behavior offers security and provides guidelines for evolving specific actions to help people.

Fifth, the use of religious practices is also another point to keep in mind while working with Spanish-American people. It is particularly important to recognize Spanish-American's dependence on God and their theory about illness causation and cure. The role of the priest in the community should also be used in planning and implementing health programs; in general, the nurse must be aware of the important role of religion and religious practitioners in the lives of the Spanish-American people.

Sixth, the nurse must consider local, social and cultural factors producing an illness, rather than focusing upon Anglo-American views of the factors that cause illness. Every cultural group generally has different kinds of stressors affecting their health state, and we must determine what these factors are and how we can ease undue stress which causes illness. In addition, the nurse must have knowledge of the local classification of illnesses and how the people currently treat the illness.

And finally, if the nurse wishes to have positive experiences with the Spanish-American people, she must occasionally visit with them in their homes and community in order to see them functioning and living in their own special community. More and more nurses will be expected to know and work with Spanish-Americans in their homes and community settings in order to be of maximum help to them. Knowing the patient in *his own cultural context* means knowing the patient in a very special and privileged way.

In sum, factors contributing to an understanding of Spanish-American behavior and their health-illness system have been presented in this chapter. The cultural context approach to understanding people is a broad and comprehensive one, which makes one realize the many variables influencing behavior. The nurse can have a positive, enjoyable, and therapeutic relationship with Spanish-American people if she gives thought to the guidelines for nursing practice outlined above.

FOOTNOTES

[1] Many of the ideas expressed in this chapter have been formulated by the author on the basis of her three years of study with Spanish-speaking families in an urban and semi-rural community in Colorado.
[2] John Burma, *Spanish-Speaking Groups in the United States*, Duke University Press, London, 1954.
[3] Bob Huber, "Verdict Strenghtens Tijerina Movement," *The Denver Post*, Sunday, Dec. 29, 1968, p. 40.

⁴Sam Schulman and Anne M. Smith, "The Concept of Health Among Spanish-Speaking Villagers of New Mexico and Colorado," *Journal of Health and Human Behavior*, Vol. 4 (1963), pp. 226-233.
⁵Arthur J. Rubel, "Concepts of Disease in Mexican American Culture," *American Anthropologist*, LXII, (October, 1960), pp. 795-814.
⁶Lyle Saunders, et al, *Handbook for Public Health Nurses*, unpublished document, Santa Fe, New Mexico, June 1964.
⁷Sam Schulman, "Rural Healthways in New Mexico," *Annals of the New York Academy of Science*. Vol. 84 (1960), pp. 950-958.
⁸Lyle Saunders, *Cultural Difference and Medical Care*, Russell Sage Foundation, New York, 1954.
⁹*Ibid.*, 377-40.
¹⁰Robert C. Hanson and Lyle Saunders, *Nurse-Patient Communication*, The Bureau of Sociological Research, Institute of Behavioral Science, University of Colorado, Boulder and the New Mexico State Department of Public Health, Santa Fe, New Mexico, 1964.
¹¹Madeleine Leininger, *Field Study Observations with Spanish-Speaking Peoples in an Urban Community, 1966-69,* unpublished report, 1969.
¹²Hansen and Saunders. *op. cit., 1964.*

SUGGESTED REFERENCES

Clark, Margaret, *Health in the Mexican-American Culture: A Community Study*, Berkeley and Los Angeles: University of California Press, 1959.

Gillin, John, "Magical Fright," *Psychiatry*, Vol. 11 (1948), 387-400.

Kiev, Ari, *Magic, Faith and Healing: Studies in Primitive Psychiatry Today*, London: The Free Press of Glencoe, Collier-Macmillan Limited, 1964.

Madsen, William, *The Mexican-American of South Texas*, New York: Holt, Rinehart and Winston, 1964.

McWilliams, Carey, *North From Mexico: The Spanish Speaking People of the United States*, Philadelphia: J. B. Lippincott Company, 1948.

Suchman, Edward, "Social Patterns of Illness and Medical Care," *Journal of Health and Human Behavior*, Vol. 6 (1965), 2-16.

9 An Adopted Vietnamese Child: A Cultural Shock

Co-Authors: Charlotte Heidema, M.S., R.N. (Nurse Therapist) and Madeleine Leininger, Ph.D., R.N.[1]

Stevie: the Adopted Child

Tired, frightened, and confused after his trip, Stevie, a three-year-old boy from Saigon, met his new parents at a busy International Airport on November 25, 1966. The press and friends of the foster parents had been waiting to welcome him. Just twenty-three hours before, Stevie's eight-year-old classificatory "sister" had taken him to a social worker's office in Saigon, South Viet Nam. The social worker had taken the small boy to a woman who later put him on a plane bound for Los Angeles. In Los Angeles, Stevie was given to a man who accompanied him on another large plane to his new city home in the Rocky Mountain area.

Until this time, Stevie's short life in Viet Nam had been fairly simple, quiet, and routine. And then, suddenly, he was moved from his familiar homeland environment, his parents, his kinsmen, and his neighborhood playmates to a noisy, fast-moving world. This boy experienced, in his own unique and silent world, cultural shock. *Cultural shock* is the bewildering experience of finding oneself suddenly in another culture which is so strikingly different from one's own that it is almost impossible to make sense out of all the unfamiliar people and things.

Back in Viet Nam, Stevie had shared his unpretentious dwelling with a large extended family group. He had been cared for by his mother and many mothering persons, e.g., his aunts, uncles, grandparents, and older siblings. These caring persons had a way of casually, calmly, and effectively caring for him without much commotion or pressure. Stevie had slept on a grass mat on the dirt floor with the rest of the family. He was bathed when necessary in a small running stream near the village, and he was fed when there was food available. His active body movements had not been restricted by lots of clothing nor bedding. In general, Stevie's physical and social environment in Viet Nam was open, free, and an integral part of the world about him. Grass, dirt, trees, and many interested persons were his friends, comfort, and protection. He had learned to know what to expect of his environment and had mastered his dealings with it fairly well.

Having lived only three years, Stevie had already learned many things. He had learned that approval was given in return for submissiveness and obedience. And since he was one of many siblings and other family members, he had learned to share what little there was and to accept the limits of what was not available. He became sensitive to others and learned to be reasonably flexible and content with life situations. Stevie's needs had been met casually as they arose, and he received no special attention or rewards. He had learned to trust the people around him and had learned by their largely non-verbal behavior what he could expect from them.

Having only lived three years, however, there were some things that Stevie had not learned. He did not know that the food in the village was not bountiful enough to supply all of the families and that as a result many families were forced to move to the city. Nor did he realize that his mother was deeply concerned about his future because he was part Vietnamese and part American. Stevie had no knowledge of his American father and had never seen him so that he had not felt the fear of being alone or the doubts of being unwanted. He had not even learned to fear American G.I.'s who came to his village and gave him candy. How was he to know that these men might come back to destroy his home? Stevie never did understand why his "sister" had taken him away from his mother and sent him to live with a strange couple in a strange place.

Stevie's New World

And now in the United States, Stevie's new home and immediate surroundings were noticeably different to him. People were moving about rapidly, bright lights were flashing, and everyone seemed to be making a lot of noise. Soon Stevie found himself being held by another strange man who was talking to him in a strange language with strange body gestures. Everyone was smiling at him. Undoubtedly Stevie must have felt that he had done something that pleased them, and sohe smiled back at them. Because he had been brought to a high mountainous environment where it was much colder than in Viet Nam, he was cold, and one could see his fragile body shivering uncontrollably.

After moving in with his new and strange adopted parents, he often found himself being held in an unfamiliar way in their arms as they moved about the house. Everything was so strange. Stevie found himself in a special room with many material objects just for him. Many of the play objects in his room were bright colors and were either very hard or very soft material. All the toys made strange noises when you handled them. Stevie was soon introduced to strange food of a different consistency, form, and taste than the food he ate in Viet Nam. He would stare at it and was afraid to eat even though he was hungry. He would eat only small portions, and frequently he would be sick afterwards.

During the first few days he watched these different-looking people talk to each other in an unintelligible language. He could not understand their gestures, talk, or behavior, and he felt very much alone and different from them. He also seemed to be looking and waiting for the rest of the family members to appear, but no one came into the house. From the outset, Stevie had a desire to go outside so he could feel the grass, see the trees, and touch other environmental objects which had always been his friends. Although he could see the trees and grass from the inside of the house, he could not get to them. It was a very strange experience. Later, he discovered that a sliding glass door was the big barrier between him and the outside world.

In the evening of the first day with his new parents, Stevie was put in a room by himself. This was a new experience—one he had never encountered in Viet Nam. The bed was raised from the floor and there were bars all around him. It was a very soft and clean bed. The room and night were dark and he was alone. Suddenly, he did not feel like smiling anymore. In his silent thoughts, he hoped that if he closed his eyes and kept quiet, and then when he opened them later, maybe everything would become familiar to him again. However, his mind and body were extremely tired, exhausted, from his confrontation with strange people, a strange house, and strange surroundings so he had no trouble going to sleep.

The Adopted Parents and Their Anticipation of a Son

Mr. and Mrs. K., the adopted parents of Stevie, did not have any other children. After waiting two years, they had decided to adopt a child that "no one else wanted." Having both worked as volunteers with retarded and underprivileged children during their college years, they had retained a strong sense of humanitarianism as well as a sense of responsibility toward children. Mr. K.

had looked forward to a boy with whom he could play and talk. Mrs. K. had preferred an infant, but conceded to have a little boy of two or three years.

The two years of marriage for Mr. and Mrs. K. had been happy and prosperous. Mr. K., a research electrician, was gone from home during the day, and occasionally he would leave for a week or two to attend a symposium or to study an aspect of his research work. Mrs. K. filled her day with her own projects such as writing, painting, and reading. Neither believed that he should sacrifice his privacy nor personal interests for the other, and in this way both had maintained a high degree of individuality and independent creativity. They had established some social relationships in the community through business, church, and club acquaintances.

Mr. and Mrs. K. had announced their plans to adopt a child to several friends, and were pleased with the publicity that accompanied their eagerness and anticipations. They were confident that they could give Stevie love, a good home with all of the conveniences necessary for his learning and growth, and opportunities far beyond the range of his imagination. And after the first few hours with their new son, they believed their dreams had become a reality.

Mr. K. was proud of Stevie's beautiful physical coordination and mastery of his body. He anticipated having him become a partner and companion on hikes and excursions. Mrs. K. had immediately responded to his openness and friendly acceptance. She enjoyed the feelings of motherliness that he evoked in her and looked forward to many experiences that would fill her need for human contact. Mr. and Mrs. K. felt that the past two years of waiting had been worthwhile, and that the future for the three of them looked hopeful and exciting.

The Family Adjustment

Stevie awoke the next morning to the strangeness and not to the familiarity he had fantasized. The flood of new stimuli and perceptions overwhelmed him. He touched, smelled, heard, saw, and tasted so many new things—and all at once. Most important, his old ways of communicating his needs and feelings were not understood by his new parents, and so he resorted to occasional temper tantrums when his basic needs were thwarted.

Stevie had never seen a toilet before and his parents' eagerness for him to use the toilet only increased his fear of it. He was afraid of the cold, hard, noisy toilet, but Mrs. K. made it clear to him that he had to learn how to use it regardless of how much it terrified him. Mrs. K., in her eagerness to show and teach him, had demanding requests for him all day, but much of the time he could not understand her. Stevie learned to follow Mrs. K. and watch her every minute because he did not want her to leave him, he was so lonely. He would follow her footsteps around the house without full awareness of what she was doing or teaching him. Mr. K., the strange new man, was gone most of the time; however, when he was home, Mrs. K. gave him a lot of attention so that Stevie had to be sneaky in getting what he wanted. Trying to get what he wanted became a kind of game. Mr. and Mrs. K. thought it would be wonderful to send Stevie to nursery school. However, each day that Stevie came home from nursery school, he seemed more troubled and distraught by the experience. After a few days with a group of strange people and strange objects, he managed to cause enough disturbance so that he did not have to return.

Stevie seemed to have his most carefree and relaxing moments when he was outside among the trees and grass—this was a familiar world to him. He would run and laugh and no one would stop him. He could feel, see, taste, and smell the things that had been familiar in his Vietnamese physical environment. It was apparent that he was very happy when he was outdoors.

More and more Stevie began to live in his own world. He would not talk and only mimicked sounds. His foster parents sent him to a speech therapist, but after several months there was no noticeable improvement in his speech. He even stopped mimicking the speech sounds of the therapist and then developed his own noises which Mrs. K. learned to associate with certain needs, moods, and desires.

Bedtime continued to be a frightening event. Many times at night he would wake up screaming. Efforts to quiet him were useless. Attempts on the part of Mr. K. to comfort Stevie seemed only to increase his terror and suspicion. Mrs. K. was the only one who could quiet him at bedtime. During the day Stevie was restless, bored, nervous, and hard to manage, but also hard to ignore. He was hyperactive and he had developed repetitive activities such as slamming a cupboard door over and over or running around in circles. He ignored his bright new toys and would show no interest in learning how to play with them.

Later Stevie began to cry frequently, and it seemed easier to the parents to leave him alone than to try and understand him or to help him; much of his behavior, however, could not be ignored. For example, whenever he was upset or excited he would run full force into the large glass door. He would do this many times in a day, and Mrs. K. had to brace herself every time it happened. Her attempts to stop him only upset him more.

Mr. K. was unsuccessful in his early attempts to engage Stevie in play or conversation, and soon his discouragement led him to avoid Stevie and to set even more distance between himself and his son. Mrs. K., on the other hand, became Stevie's primary focus and interest. She developed her own routine, adapting to his behavior mainly by catering to his needs and protecting him from the scrutiny of outsiders. She was not, however, getting the full maternal satisfactions she had initially desired from her son.

One year and a half after his arrival from Viet Nam, Stevie was a changed boy. His eyes were blank and seldom met the eyes of another person. He was excitable and could be controlled only temporarily through stern commands. He did not talk or play with other children. He could not dress himself and needed constant reminders to use the bathroom. He showed signs of varying moods during the day. At times he was angry, sad, and destructive, and then he would express affection and act as if he were happy. One could feel that his behavior came out of his own silent but active inner world.

The frustration, disappointment, and helplessness that Mr. and Mrs. K. experienced finally brought them to a child developmental clinic. Stevie was seen by a number of professional staff members, and was soon diagnosed as acute schizophrenia and a mentally retarded child. At that time, the distraught parents acknowledged that they hoped Stevie could be institutionalized. Their friends and neighbors had begun to comment about Stevie's bizarre behavior. Mr. and Mrs. K. were disappointed and reluctant to face what they perceived as the serious social stigma of having a child who was defective—both mentally and physically.

Nurse-Family Relationship As Experienced by the Nurse Therapist

It was in June, 1968, that I met this family. At the time, I was a graduate student in psychiatric nursing. Undaunted by Stevie's poor prognosis or by the child psychiatrist's guarded hopes for any results from intensive therapy, I began seeing the family in their home on a weekly basis. I visited them, at the request of the clinic psychiatrist, primarily to offer support to the parents while Stevie was in play therapy.

Throughout the course of an on-going experience with Stevie and his foster parents, I became painfully aware of my personal prejudices and values through a self-supervision process. I recognized in myself these biases and deep concerns: How could these parents do this to such a healthy, robust little fellow? Did they scapegoat him to resolve their own marital difficulties and personal conflicts? Why had they chosen such an innocent, naive victim to meet their own needs? They had assumed the responsibility of parenting this child and now, when it was probably too late, they wanted professional help. Why had they uprooted Stevie from his native home and land? Would not it have been better to leave him with his mother and his family in his own country?

It took several months for me to understand the situation and to partially resolve some of these questions. After weeks of observation, analysis, and supervision, and the sharing of experiences with the family members at mealtime and naptime, in play in the backyard, and during a shopping trip with the family, I began to understand some of their feelings and mine. Frustration, helplessness, anger, confusion, and an attitude of hopelessness were some of the feelings that had produced despair in this family. Only after accepting their feelings and understanding their dilemma, could I begin to offer support and assurance.

I began to realize that the lack of planning and guidance for the parents who had chosen a child from another culture had led to serious problems. Their expectations, confusion, and misunderstanding of the child led to much disappointment and frustration. Consequently, anger and guilt ensued and these led to an avoidance of the child and a denial of the child's problems. The barriers had grown rapidly between the parents and their adopted child until the only recourse they could accept was separation from him. The problem seemed unsurmountable, the mixture of emotions was too frightening, and the road of therapy seemed far too long and uncertain. In January of 1969, Mr. and Mrs. K. decided they did not want to jeopardize their chances of having a happy family, and so they took Stevie out of therapy and placed him in a foster home. The foster home was only a temporary placement until there would be an opening for him at an institution for retarded children.

My work with this family was a difficult experience. Overcoming personal prejudices and values was a necessary step toward a supportive and nonjudgmental approach to the family. Initially, my hopes of helping the family were high, but soon I recognized what had happened to the child and I knew the amount of time it would undoubtedly take to help him. It would also take considerable time to support the parents and to help them to accept Stevie and their mixed feelings about him. After Mr. and Mrs. K. had made the decision to give up Stevie, I was left with deep feelings of disappointment and failure. I had formed a close relationship with Stevie and our mutual trust enabled us to work through the termination phase. I was not satisfied with what had happened to the child and the parents, and so I pursued a more academic and objective evaluation of this situation, considering in particular what might have been done differently, and what implications this situation could have for parents and nurse clinicians in the future.

About this time, I was also beginning a seminar entitled "Nursing and Anthropology," which I hoped would give me a good opportunity to explore in depth both the cultural and nursing dimensions related to Stevie and Mr. and Mrs. K.

A Comparison of the Two Cultures

A comparison of the cultural differences of the parents and the child became the focus of my study. In my search of the literature regarding cultural aspects of inter-country adoptions, I found only limited information pertaining to this topic, and none that related specifically to the transcultural adoption of a child from Viet Nam to America. My next step was to study the complex Vietnamese culture, make inferences from this data, and develop an appropriate nursing care plan of therapy. In studying the cultural factors relevant to this case, I needed to study the specific culture of South Viet Nam which Stevie had left, and take into account the fact that he had come from the lower rural class.

Culture History Aspects and the Cultural Context. Geographical, social, cultural, and educational environments vary throughout Viet Nam; however, in a general portrait of the people one can see differences between the rural and urban peoples. The old history of the Vietnamese is fascinating. It is packed with a long record of political conquerors and reconquering experiences, different kinds of Chinese rulers, economic achievements, a strong drive to preserve the Chinese culture and technical knowledge, and a perpetual struggle to maintain their own identity as a distinct cultural group. The Vietnamese people had beautiful indigenous art, well-made homes, skillfully cast weapons, domesticated animals and wheat and millet crops as early as the 12th century B.C.

From 940 to 1400 A.D. the Vietnamese lived mainly in the northern part of the country and lived under a relatively stable and efficient government strong enough to withstand Chinese aggression and incursions from Cambodia. About the middle of the 15th century the Vietnamese began their "march to the South." This marked the beginning of internal difficulties which separated the country into many political divisions. It was only after 1802 that the country regained its territorial unity, and experienced the greatest military achievements in the history of their country. Up until the early part of the 20th century, Viet Nam had had many rulers and dynasties which led the people to become deferent and acquiesing to the ruling power. Later, the South Vietnamese people were exposed to French, Japanese, and American domination. Throughout their history the Vietnamese people have been exposed to a variety of rulers and to threats from within and outside.[2]

Sociocultural, Economic, and Kinship Factors. The rural Vietnamese are timid, humble, and simple peasants who lead a horticultural and fishing existence. They have learned to work hard for their superiors, but to preserve at all cost their cultural values and their identity. They have a high degree of sensitivity to their land and to each other, and they are very much a part of their physical environment. These peasant people are not apathetic to strangers; on the contrary, they are very curious about foreigners. They do, however, expect strangers to be warm, receptive, and kind in response to their good will and fairness to others. Rural Vietnamese maintain a timid sophistication, which is an integrated response within their own cultural etiquette. Modesty and indirectness are important in relating to others.

The rural Vietnamese are more traditional than the urban people, a fact which has contributed to a sizeable gap in economic levels. In contrast to the luxurious dwellings of some Vietnamese in the cities, the rural people live in thatch homes. These thatch homes characteristically have a dirt floor, no sanitary facilities, and no running water or electricity. The Vietnamese peasants are predominately skilled rice cultivators or fishermen. Among this peasantry group there remains the strong influence of Confucianism, the principal religion that has pervaded the history of the Vietnamese. This traditional religion is a source of attitudes and values which guide the people.[3]

Family and kinsman are extremely important to the Vietnamese villager; in fact, the family is more important than the individual. South Vietnamese families are respected and important to the well being and social development of every individual. A Vietnamese learns to rely upon his own family and their ties to the larger community, and to other kinship groups. The family which is the unit of ownership, production, and management, is not limited to a nuclear family unit, but is extended to include the larger household of an older man and wife with their married sons, daughter-in-law and grandchildren. Although family ties reach out, as they have for thousands of years in this culture, to a wide group of relatives with the most tenuous bonds of kinship, the crux of family loyalty is filial piety which commands children to honor their father and mother, to do everything to make them happy, and to worship their memory after their death. This commandment provides strength, stability, and continuity to the large family group composed of all those descending from a claimed male ancestor. Immediate family relationships are more influential than are broader sociocultural relationships.

The pattern of respect that a child has for his father, and that, by analogy, the father has for his elders and for those in authority over him, is deeply ingrained in every Vietnamese from earliest childhood. To most Vietnamese, filial piety and respect for the father's lineage is not abstract theory but a law of nature pervading all natural relationships. To them, this attitude is inborn —a child naturally feels respect for his father. Family loyalty inextricably binds the individual to hearth and home. For most Vietnamese, not only emotional security but economic well-being depend upon the family. The individual Vietnamese will compromise most obligations in the interest of family ties and family unity. It is probably difficult for us to understand the power and importance of the family and kinsmen to the Vietnamese.

Vietnamese Socialization Processes. Early childhood is a relatively free and unrestrained period of life for the Vietnamese. Mutually supporting forces are brought to bear in training the child. First, the parents expect that the child will submit to their guidance without questioning, argument, or hesitation. Back-talk from a child is shocking to adults, and marked independence is discouraged. Children must ask permission of parents for whatever they do, and keep them closely informed of their activities and whereabouts. The main responsibility for the child's socialization rests with the parents; however, an array of extended kinsmen are active agents in making the child a respected and wanted person in the society. The older brothers and sisters play an important part and command respect from the child. Even the family ancestors play an important role in the process of socialization. In the traditional Vietnamese household, the child becomes keenly aware of these unseen senior kinsmen. He comes to feel their presence and learns that they are deeply involved in his life. The child learns to respect, fear, and admire them from the attitude of his parents, who stress their strength and virtues. The child is urged to follow the example of his ancestors for moral, ethical, and social guidance.

The typical Vietnamese feels strongly that it is everyone's duty at all times to maintain an even temper and to be just and fair to all men. He places great emphasis on self-control, rarely shows his feelings, and prefers to avoid expressions of disagreement which might irritate or offend. A loud voice, or a public display of arrogance, anger, or affection, is considered coarse and unmannerly. The Vietnamese has been called a slave to etiquette. In a given situation, it is more important and admirable to adjust to a principle of behavior than to maintain firm adherence to an immutable principle of morality. The Vietnamese have a proverb which states that the supple bending reed survives storms which break the strong but unyielding oak. To the Vietnamese, no position is irretrievable; no commitment is final.

American Culture and Socialization Values. In contrast to the culture of rural South Viet Nam, Mr. and Mrs. K., Stevie's new parents, belonged to the upper-middle class western urban American culture. In their culture the mean economic level is considerably higher than in Viet Nam. Mr. and Mrs. K.'s social group was comprised of people who belonged to professional organizations and worked in or owned small businesses.

As discussed earlier in this book, the American culture stresses such values as achievement, success, education, independence, and a strong sense of individualism. Emphasis is placed on the accumulation of material goods to verify one's success and social status. Christianity and the Protestant work ethic are powerful influences on the people, as is the emphasis on maintaining a pioneering and adventurous spirit. Materialism manifest in a variety of technical facilities and conveniences has provided a guide to living. A typical living room of a family in the American culture may contain a stereo, a television, an air conditioner, lamps, a table, chairs, a sofa, wall-to-wall carpeting, bookshelves, paintings, windows, drapes, plants, and sundry personal treasures. Other rooms in the home are equipped with special devices to enhance the values of cleanliness, comfort, beauty, and efficiency.

The family structure in the American culture also contrasts markedly with the extended kinship system of Viet Nam. The nuclear family has the predominant place in the lives of Americans. It is composed of the husband, wife, and their children. The nuclear family is relatively isolated, and one's ties with relatives are often fragmented and superficial. More importance is placed on social and occupational relationships outside of the nuclear family. Mr. and Mrs. K.'s contacts with close and distant kinsmen were infrequent and of limited social significance. Emotional ties within the nuclear American family center around common experiences within the family group and a desire to meet the needs of each individual within the family unit.

The American social structure is highly complex. Educational, religious, legal, political, and economic institutions regulate the activities of people. Fast transportation and mobility allow the individuals and families to move about in their environment with ease. Recreational activities and the joys of nature are largely institutionalized and found primarily in such areas as parks, zoos, and specific recreational areas.

Certain expectations derived from the American social structure, cultural values, and the family structure, are reflected in its child-rearing practices. In contrast with the Vietnamese norm, early and fairly rigid training is practiced in the homes of the American upper-middle class. Early toilet training is highly rewarded. The child is expected to adjust to social situations and to the expectations of each parent. The full use of educational toys and the pressure to perform independently are examples of the stress placed on the child towards achievement and independence. Rewards are given for ambition, aggression, and competitive supremacy. Generally, the parents are non-indulgent and fairly severe in the socialization of the child, and use intellectual talk and play to help him understand the world about them.

Typically, the father in this culture is away from home for most of the day, and so primary emphasis centers upon the mother-child relationship. The child soon learns that his mother is an individual whom he must trust, but he also learns early to meet his own needs and assert his own individuality. The child is also encouraged to exert himself and to value self-expression and freedom. From infancy, the child learns to demand his own individual rights and privileges, and he often gets what he wants and needs through making himself heard. This high emphasis upon the individual in socialization is in marked contrast with the group emphasis in Viet Nam.

Inferences From the Cultural Data Regarding Stevie

Undoubtedly the rigid, achievement-oriented, independent, and somewhat compulsive atmosphere that Stevie encountered in his new American home was in shocking contrast to the relaxed, indulgent, and flexible home situation in Viet Nam. In addition, the assertive role he was expected to play in America was the opposite of the submissive behavior he had been expected to exhibit as a Vietnamese child. Probably one of the most shocking discoveries was that

Stevie was accustomed to having several mother figures and then suddenly he had only one, Mrs. K. Although Mrs. K. was attentive to Stevie, at times she would retreat into her own world to do painting and writing. Stevie must have wondered what had happened to his mother and must have felt some rejection when no one was readily and continually available to him. At three years of age, it would be difficult to perceive this drastic multiple mother separation as anything but traumatic and extremely painful to this active and alert boy.

Then, too, the father-son relationship in Viet Nam was different from the father-son relationship in America. Before, Stevie had responded to his Viet Nam uncle as a figure to be respected and obeyed without question, while his nurturant and companionship needs had been met primarily by females. Now his American father wanted an intimate and giving relationship with him. His culturally-oriented respect and awe for "fathers" turned into fear and panic with Mr. K.'s behavior, especially when the paternal demands for interaction and affection became too strong. Stevie responded with terror whenever Mr. K. put him to bed and tucked him in for the night. Besides the fact that his new father assumed a different role than the one which was expected in his native culture. In addition, Stevie had never before slept in a bed raised from the floor and in a totally dark room. He must have been terrified to experience such drastic changes in his sleeping environment. But most important, he had never before slept alone in a bed. It was a strange and frightening experience not to feel the closeness of other persons with him throughout the night when Stevie had slept with as many kinsmen as six to eight on the floor of his Viet Nam hut. Stevie had not been accustomed to interacting with strange and unknown people; he was used to being surrounded by familiar kinsman. His sudden exposure to many new people in the nursery school and in speech therapy was another frightening and terrifying experience.

Then one must pause and wonder about differences in sensory experiences for Stevie. The sudden exposure to a strange and wide variety of sensations must have strained his perceptual input and produced a sensory overload. Evidently, this sensory overload led to distortions and compulsive behavior in order for him to maintain a sense of security midst the strangeness of his new world. For example, his expression of frustration by banging into the glass door was evidence of his confusion and the feeling of being cut off from the outside world. The glass doors and windows tantalized his desires, but frustrated his goal of getting outside. Also, the toilet was unnatural to him. To have water destroy objects so quickly and completely was not a part of his past experience, and threatened his own existence. Cleanliness was a new concept, and he must have interpreted a midday change of clothing in the bathroom as a form of punishment. The opportunity to get dirty and stay dirty was not permitted in the American socialization practices.

In light of these and many other changes to which Stevie was expected to adjust in a strange and lonely culture, one must first raise the critical question and ask if Stevie was actually "mentally retarded," or was his more a situation of "serious cultural conflicts." From all observational and biographical data, Stevie was viewed as a very alert, bright, and sensitive child in his early development, but during the first two years he was in America, he was changing his behavior noticeably. The constant exposure to strange people, their ways and stresses were telling on Stevie. He could not make cognitive sense out of most of his experiences and gradually he withdrew and became ill. Furthermore, cultural skewing could have easily occurred in the testing procedures which did not examine how Stevie was responding to the test stimuli from his native cultural viewpoint. There were probably many incidences of misinterpretation of the responses to fit American perceptions of stimuli and not Stevie's early cultural frame of reference. Unfortunately, none of the professional staff were knowledgeable about cultural ways of the Vietnamese people, and so no one evaluated the tests in light of these aspects. Thus a *cultural disorder*, rather than a genetic disorder, brain damage, or mental retardation, appears to have been the relevant diagnosis. Interpreting Stevie's behavior to a vague organic condition which was not validated and inferring behavior which did not take into account the many cultural conflicts which Stevie experienced appeared to be what had happened in the analysis of Stevie's behavior.

Stevie had to cope with a tremendous number of changes, and so he gradually discovered that social withdrawal and ritualistic behavior were ways to handle confusion in a new culture. Analyzing these life experiences from a cultural viewpoint, a different plan of intervention could have been used with Stevie and can be used by nurses and health professionals as a guide in future transcultural adoptions.

Nursing Plan for Future Situation like Stevie's Case

A plan of intervention or of anticipatory guidance would begin very early when parents mention their desire to adopt a child from another culture. Hopefully, such a plan could be put into effect at the time the parents first talk to a professional person about adoption and before they submit an application for a child. If the parents do not follow the regular channels for adoption, the plan should not be abandoned, but a more intensive plan should be initiated at the time that the child is brought into the home.

Before a child from another culture actually comes to his foster parents, a knowledgeable and open discussion about cultural differences should be staged so the new parents will not be blind to the facts. Then a system of support should be made available for the parents. This system should be comprised of various key people. First of all, the agencies for adoption should be resources for information and education. Too often, representatives of these agencies are seen only as screening agents, and the parents are inhibited from talking thoroughly about their expectations. Unfortunately, emphasis is placed on physical interests, psychological motivations (individual and family), and economic stability, and seldom are cultural factors and areas of cultural conflicts discussed. Throughout the history of adoption, a system has evolved which has proven quite adequate in determining physical and psychological compatibility, but much more work must be done in determining the cultural differences and compatibilities between parents and child.

Another source of support would be the families who have already adopted a child from the same culture. These parents would have a wealth of information readily available for expectant parents. They could share their successes and failures, their helpful hints, and words of caution. Forming an ongoing group or club of these parents would offer an immediate available resource and would provide a setting in which parents could discuss their problems.

Besides working with professional agencies and other parents, the parents themselves should be actively involved in an educational program. Crucial areas to be studied should include the cultural background of the child, the implications of a sudden and traumatic separation, communication techniques, and exercises in picking up cue behavior. Again, the availability of a group of foster parents would enhance the project. The nurse clinician, who has been at ease with teaching pregnant mothers, could initiate and conduct these groups with expertise, provided she herself had been adequately instructed in the areas of group process, cultural background factors, and sociocultural changes.

The initial phase of preparation would be aimed toward the development of realistic expectations. From the use of supportive resources and knowledge of the child's background, the parents would have attained a degree of comfortableness and some feeling of competence at the time of the child's arrival. This type of preparation would allow the parents to remain involved in the realistic situation, and would prevent them from withdrawing or resorting to escapist maneuvers.

When the child arrives, the parents should be involved enough to make necessary adjustments that will accommodate the child's cultural and social differences and help him cope with his immediate emotional crisis. Some practical changes may be needed for the initial period of the child's adjustment. Using Stevie's experience as an example, one can think of some changes that would have facilitated his cultural transition. First, the amount of physical stimuli could have been reduced, keeping his surroundings as simple and familiar as possible. Removing the television and stereo, covering the picture window with drapes, and offering him familiar food with familiar ritual are a few examples. Mr. and Mrs. K. might have considered eating on the floor with Stevie, or sleeping on the floor in his bedroom, had they known that it would have made Stevie feel more at home. Parents should try to remain alert and sensitive to the child's reaction to his separation from his own home and his adjustment problems in a new culture. Ideally, the child should have a few old and dear items from the past in his possession. These items could help bridge the gap somewhat between past and present. Also, a few familiar words spoken in the native language would be very helpful, as there is a very close tie between language, behavior, and culture. The parents should anticipate that any separation for a period of time has a potential traumatic aspect. An event such as bedtime should be handled carefully. The child should not be left with the feeling that he is being abandoned since at any time this will reawaken all of his fears and uncertainties. Because of his anxiety, he will be seeking much assurance and security and should be given extra time and attention until he is more comfortable. Clinging and tagging behind are means of confirming physical nearness, and should be recognized and tolerated by the parents.

If indicated, the child should be allowed to regress somewhat and less emphasis should be given to the achievement of specific development tasks during the initial adjustment period. One practical consideration in Stevie's case would have been to delay toilet training until he showed interest and was adjusted to his strange environment. One could respond to his desires for fondling or affection, but not make demands from him in toilet training. One could also delay new experiences such as taking him to nursery school or playing with complicated strange toys, until he was more familiar with the people and his surroundings. Demands made of Stevie should have been simple, understandable, concrete, and limited, until he could achieve success with one or two and comfortably move on to others.

If the child is not accustomed to an intense parent-child relationship, this should be diluted to fit his needs. Inviting a few interested friends or relatives to share the first week or two might have been beneficial for both parents and Stevie as the presence of friendly and warm people coming and going would have simulated Stevie's home setting of many kinsmen around him.

Throughout the initial period, the parents should be alert to cues that the child is giving. An example with Stevie was his natural and spontaneous interest in the outdoors and the frustration he exhibited on not being able to reach the outdoors. At the first indication of frustration, the parents could have removed the irritating stimulus and replaced it with something that pleased or satisfied him. In this situation, it would have been helpful if the parents spent more time outdoors with Stevie—a natural and familiar place to him.

After the child has successfully adapted to his new environment, the parents should be aware of differences between their values and those of the child. They should be keenly perceptive in identifying areas of conflict and in assessing the child's readiness to move into new areas. For example, Mr. and Mrs. K.'s system of rewards for Stevie tried to ellicit aggressive and intelligent behavior from him. With guidance in developing their skills of observation and awareness, they could have modified their established norms to incorporate Stevie's differences. Rewards would have probably been effective in shaping his behavior if they had been offered in a simple and direct way in the form of a reward. For example, Mrs. K. might have offered Stevie a warm hug when he put a toy puzzle together. Spontaneous social rewards of casualness and warmth are important to a child adjusting to a new culture.

Some difficult areas could not have been modified but could have been accepted and worked through. Two major problems were the parents' altered sense of obligation and the child's fantasies about adoption. The adoptive mother's reaction and disappointment to a nonsuccessful adoption was probably more traumatic than for a natural mother who had a child become ill. The adopted mother had long-anticipated hopes to express her motherly interests and these hopes and desires did not fully materialize. Then, too, the child's own fantasies about finding parents and an environment in which he would feel secure and wanted must be considered. How did the child feel about having strange adopted parents? These are two big problem areas which warrant serious thought.

The nurse clinician must take her cues from the parents and child as to the positive and negative feelings and responses to adoption. The degree of involvement of the nurse therapist must be based on her continued assessment of the child-parent adjustment process. Intervening must be a constructive and sensitive response to both the adopted parents and the child's needs. The nurse's professional judgment and knowledge must guide her in her activities with the family and much of her role will depend on the parent's perception of her and their needs. Most important, the nurse therapist should function as a person who is willing to explore stressful relationships and to help the child and parents examine these stresses and behavior potentialities together.

The above account of Stevie was a true one with only slight modifications to safeguard the identity of the persons. It was, indeed, a cultural shock for Stevie, for his adopted parents, and for the nurse clinician to discover what occurred in a relatively short period of time. The consequences were not what had been anticipated, and so one must ask, what would have happened had Stevie remained in his native Vietnamese culture? Furthermore, one must ask whether the picture would have been different had the professional staff understood the cultural differences. From the nurse clinician's perspective, the consequences would have been different had she been more knowledgeable about cultural factors influencing the patient's behavior. The crux of the difficulty in this case study lay in the cultural differences between the Vietnamese and American ways of life and professional ways of responding or not responding to Stevie's special needs and stresses.

As the nurse clinician becomes knowledgeable and sensitive to measures in preventing illness, knowledge of cultural differences will be necessary to help the nurse discover cultural conflicts that can precipitate illness states. This kind of knowledge came too late for the nurse clinician helping the child in this case; however, from a retrospective view she learned what to be alert to in the future.

FOOTNOTES

Charlotte Heidma was the nurse therapist for Stevie in this case study. Dr. Leininger collaborated with her in writing the article and helped her to retrospectively analyze this situation after Miss Heidma had worked with the patient and his adopted parents. This collaborative article emerged from the seminar entitled "Anthropology and Nursing."

SUGGESTED REFERENCES

[2]*Helping and Developing the Health Program of Viet Nam,* Annual Report, Public Health Division, United States Operations Mission, Viet Nam, July 1, 1960-June 30, 1961.

[3]*U.S. Army Area Handbook for Viet Nam,* Department of Army Pamphlet No. 550-40, Washington, D.C.: Superintendent of Documents, U.S. Government Printing Office, September, 1962.

[4]Nguyen Van Thuan, *An Approach to Better Understanding of Vietnamese Society: A Primer for Americans,* Michigan State University, Vietnam Advisory Group, Saigon, Vietnam, June, 1962.

[5]Lloyd W. Woodruff, *The Study of a Vietnamese Rural Community—Administrative Activity, II.* With Annex by Nguyen Xuan Dao, *Village Government in Viet Nam: A Survey of Historical Development,* Michigan State Vietnam Advisory Group, May 1960.

10 Health Institutions as Cultural and Social Systems

Health institutions as cultural and social systems have become the recent focus of interest for social and health scientists. In recent years, health personnel have been exposed to various theories, concepts, and research findings regarding health institutions. Although there are many kinds of health institutions, the major focus in this chapter will be on the hospital; however, several concepts and theories presented here will have some relevance to other health institutions and community health agencies.

Understanding of the hospital as a cultural and social system, rather than a mere physical structure to treat sick people, has opened the door for many new ideas about patients and staff who live and interact together in a hospital. In fact, the exposure of health professionals to system behavior and system health practices has provided a whole new area of thinking and research. The nurse who has acquired this new approach to the understanding of sick and well people will be able to modify her individual single-patient approach in order to consider situations in which individuals and groups stay well or become ill in the hospital. The focus on cultural and social system behavior in hospital settings is forcing intrapsychic-oriented staff members to look now at extra-psychic factors influencing the patient's illness, recovery, and general attitude towards others.

The emphasis on health institutions as dynamic system

forces in health behavior is not only becoming a popular professional topic, but an important one to understand and help people who enter a hospital. Unfortunately, health personnel who have a limited understanding of system behavior are struggling to understand the meaning and relevance of the hospital as a social system. Nurses are among these health personnel who are eager to obtain a comprehensive picture of and scientific facts about social system behaviors of patients and staff. Such an understanding is offering new approaches to patient care and new ideas about the role of the nurse in maintaining or modifying system behavior in order to help patients recover.

Basic Definitions of Social and Cultural Systems

Fundamental to an understanding of system behavior is the need to understand the word "system." A *system* is *an assemblage of parts, persons, or objects that are united by some form of order (or relationships) and that show signs of being interdependent in their vital functioning as an organized unit or whole.* Each phrase of this definition is packed with meaning and should be carefully examined. Granted, there are many kinds of systems that would fit this definition. For example, one can speak of a telephone system, a solar system, a communication system, a health system, and so on. However, every system should meet the criteria implied in the above definition, i.e.: 1) the system must be an assemblage of persons (or objects); 2) the persons or objects must be united by some form or order or relationships; 3) the persons or objects must show signs of being interdependent; 4) they must tend to function as an organized unit or whole.

A *social system* refers to *an assemblage of people united by some form of regular interaction in which members show sets of behavior which are independent in function and yet, these behaviors are interrelated for the optimal functioning of the whole unit.* Social systems are viewed as functional units, in that groups of people interact with one another and show signs that all the groups in a defined system are interdependent and generally strive to function toward common goals or objectives. Individuals functioning in a system tend to reveal action patterns that are interrelated and interdependent.

Interrelatedness and interdependence are two key concepts in social system behavior. Although a wide variety of people work and interact together in a health institution, they all have some implicit or explicit common goals. A hospital staff, for instance, works together to help patients get well and maintain their defined health status. In other kinds of institutions, such as health agencies, schools of nursing, and child guidance centers, related goals can also be identified. Every institution has its unique patterns or styles of interaction, as well as its own degree of being interrelated and interdependent. Anthropologists and sociologists seek to discover and explain institutional systems and how they influence people's behavior. Essentially, social system behavior focuses upon the *patterns of interaction within institutions and the ways the group members are interconnected and interdependent.*

A *cultural system* is concerned with the normative beliefs, values, and action patterns of a designated group of people who show signs of being interrelated and interdependent. With a cultural system, the major focus is upon the *norms* of a particular group of people in an institution and how these norms regulate the group's actions, interactions, and beliefs. It is also concerned with symbolic and nonsymbolic expressions of behavior, and how these expressions increase or decrease the degree of relatedness among group members. *Norms*, or *rules of behavior*, are important determinates of cultural systems, and so the social scientist examines them in depth.

In studying a cultural system, one obtains data on the norms of behavior of a particular institution or group and data on how the people function in relation to their special rules of behavior. As one might suspect, some groups tend to conform rigidly to prescribed norms while others may deviate considerably from them. The degree of conformity or nonconformity to system norms provides many clues about the patterns of interaction of the people and gives clues to predict what people will do in the system when subjected to stress and crises. Some subgroups in a system diverge considerably from the norm behavior of the total group, and this may be a sign of their desire to change the norms of the system or to rebel against certain kinds of behavior found in the system. A wide variety of patterns related to normative and non-normative behavior can be identified in social systems. As social scientists study system behavior, some tend to concentrate on concrete and descriptive statements about a system; whereas other scientists may strive for highly abstract formulations—*i.e.*, its members' abstract and symbolic beliefs and practices about system behavior. The more abstract the formulations are about system behavior, the more difficult it will be for the nurse unprepared in the social science field to understand system behavior. This unprepared nurse should, however, strive to obtain a rudimentary descriptive account of system behavior in order to give her a fresh and broad view of the patient and staff's behavior from both a social and cultural system perspective.

Formal and Informal Systems. Cultural and social systems are also studied as *formal* and *informal* systems of behavior. In considering *formal system* behavior, one looks for the sanctioned, well-known, prescribed, and generally visible patterns of interaction within a system. In considering *informal system* behavior one is concerned with interaction patterns that tend to be covert, casual, less-sanctioned, and non-prescribed by the formal channels of administration. Informal system behavior is generally spontaneous. Let us turn to some examples of formal and informal system behavior.

Staff ward conferences held in hospital settings are an example of a formal system of behavior. Generally, staff conferences are held regularly each morning, with professional and nonprofessional staff attending to discuss patient needs and problems and to plan care strategies for the day. These meetings are prescribed by persons in authority roles, and the staff is expected to attend the meetings each day. In contrast, a spontaneous staff meeting held at a coffee shop away from the hospital would constitute an informal system of behavior. Staff nurses may come together for a cup of coffee in the morning and soon find themselves discussing many weighty staff problems and making decisions about what they would like to do as a group to improve patient care; their ideas may then be brought to the formal meeting where action is taken to affect these changes. It is not uncommon to find that group ideas discussed in informal situations have become sanctioned and formally recognized at a later time. Informal system behavior is of considerable relevance as it is often the source of emerging new system norms, of ways to achieve new system goals, and of ways to change determining formal systems of behavior. Many social scientists are currently directing their energies toward a study of informal systems which, they contend, offer significant clues about normative behavior changes in a system and the factors contributing to the changes or the stability of a particular system. Informal system behavior also offers clues about new leadership and followship patterns and the source of interpersonal difficulties in the system. Both informal and formal system data, however, are essential for a comprehensive understanding of system behavior and they tend to complement one another.

Open and Closed Systems. As one moves in and out of different kinds of systems, one soon detects that systems are either *open* or *closed*. An *open system* refers to a group of people within a designated setting who readily permit the assimilation of new people into the system and maintain an open and accepting attitude toward unfamiliar ideas, modes of behavior, and actions. In other words, persons functioning in an open system tend to permit new ideas and different action patterns to enter their system. In contrast, a *closed system* refers to a group of people who do not tend to facilitate, encourage, or accept new members, ideas, and practices into their system. Closed systems are essentially restrictive as to whom and/or what they will allow to enter their system. One generally finds that the norms of closed systems are well defined, highly valued, and inflexible; on the other hand, persons in an open system tend to be willing to accommodate diverse ideas and members, and willing to recruit new members and even change their own patterns of recruiting. Closed and open systems are fascinating units for study and have much relevance to nurses who can promote either closed or open systems by their actions and beliefs.

Macro and Micro Systems. A *micro sociocultural system* refers to a small number of people who constitute a group and are interrelated and interdependent. For example, one can view the family or the ward of a particular hospital as two kinds of micro systems. As the term implies, a micro system is a small, readily identifiable, and clearly delineated unit of human interaction. Accordingly, a *macro sociocultural system* is a large and complex network of people who are interrelated and interdependent. Hospitals, universities and communities are macro systems. Macro systems are difficult to study because one usually finds many complex and ambiguous relationship patterns that have obscure relationships to other groups in the system. It is the author's contention that nurses without special preparation in anthropology or sociology should leave macro systems to be studied and analyzed by qualified and experienced social scientists. However, nurses who have had social science courses in their nursing programs can generally understand and appreciate the findings about complex macro systems, and often can suggest ways to implement recommendations derived from the findings. One can predict that nurses in the near future will become more involved in studying different kinds of micro social and cultural systems in order to understand and plan for better care to patients. They, too, will realize the tremendous impact of institutional system behavior upon the patient's recovery and the staff's performance and attitudes. Recently, nurses with doctoral preparation in the social sciences have been studying system behavior, and find it rewarding and informative. Non-nurse studies of social and cultural health systems of institutions and of communities have been made by Caudill,[2] Cummings,[3] Stanton and Schwartz,[4] Goffman,[5] von Mering and King,[6] and others. The work from these authors has stimulated nurses to think in new directions.

Three Dimensions for Studying Sociocultural Systems

In seeking to find ways to understand aspects of social and cultural systems, the author has identified three important subsystem dimension to study and analyze these systems. Although these three dimensions are closely interrelated, they can be used as separate analytical units to examine sociocultural systems. The dimensions of study are: (1) a normative subsystem, (2) a practice subsystem, and (3) an interpersonal subsystem. Each of these dimensions could be applied to macro and micro, formal and informal, or closed and open systems. These three dimensions influence one another, but may operate fairly independently.

First, the *normative subsystem* refers to the explicit and implicit norms of a system which govern a group's behavior. In studying a normative system, one is concerned with the *"should be"* or *"ought to be"* behavior of people—the "believed-in" and expected ways in which people act or think. As one observes normative systems, one finds there are norms which explicitly or implicitly indicate what is prescribed or proscribed. The prescribed norms are those which define what one must do, whereas the proscribed norms say what one should not do. For example, in hospital A the nursing staff is prescribed (or expected) to report on duty fifteen minutes before the nursing staff change, in order to get a report on the patients from the staff leaving at a designated time. In this same hospital, the nurses have a proscriptive norm that their nursing notes are not to be hour-by-hour accounts of patients' behavior, but rather are to consist of a concise summaries of the patients' behavior during an eight-hour period. These norms are explicit because they are known to all the staff and the staff is expected to follow them. They serve as guides and directives of behavior. An example of an implicit norm is the custom that nurses should share their problems and conflicts with their nursing supervisor at coffee break time. Implicit norms are seldom put in writing or made explicit, yet one knows by certain cues of behavior what one is expected to do. A normative subsystem, then, is concerned with the *believed-in* and *should-be* modes or rules of behavior that exist among a designated group of people. Both explicit and implicit rules of normative behavior can be identified.

Second, there is the *practice subsystem*, which refers to the *actual performance* of a group of people in an institution. The practice subsystem reveals what people in an institution do, think, and believe. Anyone can observe the actual performance of individuals and groups in the institution. The practice subsystem is concerned with the manifest behavior of people, i.e., their performance of tasks, activities, functions, and roles in a particular setting. It reveals what people do and what they do not do in given situations. For example, the practice subsystem discloses whether or not the professional nurse talks with patients about their problems and concerns. It reveals whether a nurse interacts frequently or infrequently with patients and with different team members regarding the patient's problems. The practice system may disclose whether or not nurse clinicians are competent in dealing with the patient's care needs, and whether or not they function in a fairly autonomous manner as nurse therapists. In sum, the practice subsystem reveals what people actually do in a sociocultural system, for it is the totality of observable performance behavior of a group or groups of people.

Third, sociocultural systems can be viewed as *interpersonal relationship subsystems*. The behavior of people in an institutional system can be observed in relation to interpersonal ties and interactional patterns of people in a particular system and their influence on individuals and groups. This is an extremely important and promising method for understanding system behavior. The nature and kind of interpersonal ties and interactional patterns determine the long-range effectiveness of any system and its basic structure. As interpersonal ties change with a system, so it also affects the normative and practice subsystems considerably. Individuals and groups tend to align themselves in interpersonal sets of relationships and some groups exert powerful political and social influences upon the total system. In fact, some strong interpersonally bonded subgroups can literally "run a system" if they maintain their strong relatedness and exert group pressures on different subgroups. It is interesting to observe how interpersonal ties develop and become strong, moderate, or extremely weak ones in a system. Some groups with strong and close interpersonal ties can remain "in power" for some time, and then suddenly another subgroup may gain strong group power and overtake the subgroup running the system. Interestingly, informal leaders who are not in legitimate or sanctioned roles by the system may "rule" the system and even be influential in removing the formal or sanctioned leader of the system. Concommitantly, subgroups in power may suddenly lose their interpersonal strength and become completely powerless and without status in the system. Such drastic shifts in interpersonal power of a system has many repercussions and can cause shifts in group morale and many other kinds of system problems.

In health institutions, interpersonal subsystems are in operation with different subgroups covertly or overtly working to gain power, status, and rewards in the system. There are aspects which resemble a viable game of "gains and losses" of interpersonal influence and power. Both positive and negative consequences are usually discernible in system behavior. For example, some individuals, through their interpersonal power may work to force certain individuals out of a system to retain a subgroup's prestige and power in the system, or they may work to keep certain people in the system for other kinds of reasons. Shifts in interpersonal ties can sometimes occur rapidly and without individuals fully realizing what has happened to them and their group. Sometimes formal leaders with noticeable neurotic and psychotic attributes become involved in disrupting interpersonal subgroup ties and these leaders often cause serious problems in maintaining a healthy and productive institutional system. Generally, it is most difficult to handle a sick and destructive leader's behavior because of the real and perceived dangers toward persons who try to establish that the leader of the system is sick or incompetent in his role. A similar situation occurs when informal leaders of a subgroup are sick and continue to disrupt the total system moving from one subgroup to another.

In the author's view, interpersonal subsystem behavior is the most important dimension to examine in the study of social systems because it influences largely the other normative and practice subsystems. To date, there are only a few studies which focus upon the static and highly dynamic processes of interpersonal ties within and between different subgroups in a system. To be sure, nurses generally know that something has changed their system, but they are not aware of what actually has happened, even though they are a part of one of the subgroups in the system. A lowering of group morale, staff turnover, and a reduction in the quality of care to patients may be a consequence of negative interpersonal subgroup behavior. At the same time, one can identify positive subgroup behavior because of satisfying and constructive interpersonal relationships in a staff subgroup. Some leaders and followers of a subgroup "click" together and are highly productive and effective in the system. Thus the kind and nature of interpersonal subsystems can literally make or break the system. It is our task as nurses to become aware of the interpersonal subsystem and learn how to maintain constructive subsystems.

How does one study and learn about these three dimensions of sociocultural systems? One of the most rewarding methods is by direct and active observation of a micro-system in a health institution. Direct observation of a group's behavior over a period of time can provide much information about system behavior. One can also study these three dimensions by direct participation in a group, such as a ward unit. Regular group discussions with others interested in the same phenomenon can help to identify and contribute to information about the social and cultural systems. Still another method of studying systems is in collaboration with a social scientist who has been observing and studying institutional groups. In health institutions where social scientists are being employed, nurses have participated in aspects of their studies to learn about features of system behavior and to benefit from the social scientist's methods and insights.

Components of Sociocultural Systems

Power, social status, prestige, role-taking, role-relinquishing, and communication are major components of system behavior.

Power is a means of influencing people in certain directions and is a significant variable in any system. Power is sought after by some individuals more than others, but practically all human beings derive satisfaction from power. Power is often used in systems to gain self-recognition, to achieve financial benefits, to control the behavior of others and to ventilate latent hostilities towards others. Observing how power is used constructively and destructively should be of interest to all nurses working in a social system. If power is used destructively, there is a need to intervene so that patients and staff can survive in the afflicted system.

Social status and *prestige* are present in health institutional systems. Social status and prestige are concerned with the positions held and the recognitions possessed by certain individuals in a system. The motives, uses, and behavioral expressions of individuals with social status and prestige vary with changing situations, groups and with time. It is interesting to observe how prestige and social status influence others and affect the behavior, aspirations, and performance of others in the system.

Role-taking and *role-relinquishing* are also present in any social and cultural system. Individuals and subgroups are generally cognizant of why they take certain roles and relinquish others. Individuals are quick to discover satisfying and less satisfying roles in an institution. Some roles offer considerable security and status, while others are tenuous and onerous. Reasons why staff members take certain roles and avoid others are important clues about health institutions and should be studied to improve the operation of systems. Roles have both dynamic and static attributes. The dynamic quality of a role leads to role changes; whereas the static quality tends to lead to role stability. Some roles have subroles and they, too, may tend to be more or less static or dynamic in nature. For example, the roles of being a female or male or of being a father, mother or sibling are *ascribed roles* and do not change much over time. In contrast, a *prescribed* role such as a grocery boy may be a dynamic role, changing frequently. In general, roles are seldom totally static or dynamic, as they have both attributes. Role theory is a subject of central importance to social anthropologists and sociologists and can be studied by the nurse in formal courses through reading the literature on the subject, or studying the topic with nurse-social scientists in different health systems.

Patterns of communication, like patterns of interaction, are found in any social and cultural system. In order for a nurse to function in a social system, she should be aware of the major patterns of communication in the system. The modes of communication may be formal in nature, that is, recognized, known, and sanctioned forms of communication. Communication may also be informal, and as such is generally casual, subtle, and spontaneous. There is also a variety of communication patterns in most sociocultural systems. For example, one may encounter a *lineal* pattern of communication, in which messages are given and received in a horizontal line. Or one may find a highly *stratified* and *hierarchial pattern* of communication, in which messages are given and received through a chain of command which goes up and down on a prescribed hierarchial ladder. These and many other kinds of communication patterns can be observed in a social system. The nurse needs to observe and study the patterns of communication within a system in order to identify how she can best communicate within the system, and to become aware of how patients and staff communicate in the same system. Practically every social and cultural system has its own distinctive dynamics and patterns of communicating. In general, nursing subsystems tend to use hierarchial patterns of communication, and hospitals, too, rely upon the stratified pattern of communication. Psychiatric hospitals and psychiatric nursing subsystems are currently exploring horizontal or lineal systems of communication and finding many positive aspects to this pattern of communication.

Conceptions and Misconceptions about Sociocultural Systems

Static and Dynamic Systems. Health practitioners who are not fully aware of the theories and concepts associated with social and cultural systems often express vague ideas and misconceptions about these systems. And, of course, health personnel who have limited knowledge about social systems may be lost in understanding them. One of the common misconceptions about sociocultural systems is that they are *static systems,* which seldom change through time and under varying circumstances. Although systems may appear static, generally they have dynamic components to them and they change with time. It is difficult to find any social or cultural system that has not changed to some extent with time. There are, however, some sociocultural systems which appear more static or resistant to change than others. In contrast, some systems seem to be constantly and noticeably changing. It is the range between static and dynamic tendencies that makes social and cultural systems interesting to study and explain. Why systems veer toward change or show limited change is often related to the nature of the group members in the system, to external and internal forces exerting pressures for change, or for a stability status, and to the interactional modes and interpersonal ties of the people in the system. The kind and amount of change in any sociocultural system varies, but practically *all* systems show changes if one carefully observes them.

A closely related common conception of system behavior is that it is extremely *abstract* and *non-specific* so that only expert social scientists can understand it. While this may be partially true, still there are aspects about any social or cultural system that can be observed and understood by a sensitive and interested person. Some social scientists analyze social systems by using highly abstract and symbolic formulations; while others use very concrete and practical low-level analysis. In general, these social scientists strive to make relevant generalizations and inferences regarding system behavior. Granted, sometimes the generalizations about system behavior are difficult to understand because they are stated in language which is quite difficult to comprehend. Nevertheless, some findings can and should be understood by professional health personnel. All system behavior is ultimately understood in terms of the concrete realities of life, and the novice in nursing who is genuinely interested in system behavior should be able to learn something about the concrete performance of interpersonal relationships in, and the normative behavior in a system.

Eufunctional and Dysfunctional Systems. Another recurrent view frequently held by health personnel is that sociocultural systems tend to be *fundamentally "sick" or "destructive."* Although social systems may be perceived to be "sick" and vary in their degree of "healthiness," it is difficult to confirm this diagnosis unless one is aware of specific criteria which can be used in judging a system "sick" or "well." One can more accurately understand systems by identifying their positive and negative functions. In addition, systems may be viewed as either "eufunctional" or "dysfunctional," to the extent that they serve the purposes or goals of an institution and have positive or negative consequences upon its members. In any system, one can identify *eufunctions* and *dysfunctions* of a system, which may be either intended or unintended, and either explicit or implicit. A hospital system may be viewed as eufunctional since it helps people retain their health status. It is dysfunctional when it seldom helps people get well and stay well. A hospital could also be viewed as dysfunctional when one finds disturbed and dissatisfied people functioning in the system over an extended period of time. In contrast, eufunctional systems tend to have a positive and healthy effect upon people. In other words, if a system is eufunctional, the people in the system seem relatively satisfied as they work toward achieving goals or purposes of the institution. Some mental and general hospitals have been described as institutions which tend to inadvertently initiate, aggravate, and/or perpetuate physical and emotional illnesses. Undoubtedly, these hospitals never intended to produce illness states of people, and yet this was the consequence of the staff and hospital climate upon the patient. When systems have been studied and their eufunctional and dysfunctional features have been identified, the next step is to work toward modifying any dysfunctional aspects. Labeling a system "sick" or "destructive" and never doing anything to try and change it is a negative approach. But one must be fully aware of the nature of the system behavior before endeavoring to change it. Admittedly, however, it is true that some systems tend to remain quite destructive to people in them without anyone's being aware of how and why they operate in this fashion.

Currently, as hospitals are being studied by social scientists for their dysfunctional and eufunctional features, there are findings in the literature which should help the nurse to understand system behavior and to provide better care to people. For example, in some hospitals and health agencies, there are specific techniques and norms which promote group solidarity and help the staff grow personally and professionally through others in their subgroups. There are, of course, systems where people have been thwarted considerably in their professional growth because of questionable group norms or, perhaps a destructive or sick leader who uses her power and sick behavior to hurt others in the system. For example, a sick and destructive leader in a top position in one hospital deliberately attacked competent staff members in order to increase her image as a powerful and controlling leader. She wished to decrease the competent staff members' abilities so that she would look better and more competent to others. This leader used a "pitting" technique by pitting one staff member against another to reduce their morale and effectiveness in working together. Unfortunately, this leader had only a limited awareness of her destructive tendencies. She was functioning in the top administrative position by virtue of the "Peter Principle," i.e., she had reached her level of incompetence as she took the top position in the hierarchial organization.[8] It was an extremely difficult and dangerous task for the staff to confront her with her behavior. Although many of the perceptive staff members were aware of her behavior, they were afraid of losing their jobs if they confronted her. The competent staff members tried to modify her behavior, but the task was too time-consuming and extensive. Silently, they left the institution as there seemed little hope for change. The hospital nursing service continued to exist, but the care to patients was poor, the staff morale was low, and there was a high turn-over of staff.

Hospitals and health agencies which function well as health care systems are known by their effectiveness not only in helping patients get well, but also in helping the staff develop professional competencies and in helping them fulfill their own growth needs. Generally, these eufunctional health systems are sensitive to the needs of the staff because they know that if staff members are frustrated and unhappy their behavior will be reflected in the quality of care to patients.

Perceptive administrators of hospitals should try to reduce the boundaries that separate their people from the main stream of society, so that the staff and patients are not subject to a peculiar or strange living and working environment. Frequently, hospital systems are quite different from the outside world, and so they often increase the stresses on patients. When the boundaries between the hospital system and the outside world are so sharp, the patient and his family must struggle to understand how to adjust to a new world. Often it is necessary that the patient change his perceptions of others, his role, and his behavior in order to get well in the hospital; consequently, when he gets ready to go home, he again changes his role and behavior in order to be accepted again into his home community. Hospital staff need to become much more aware of the differences between the hospital and the patient's home and community so that they can help with this problem. Some hospitals are trying today to reproduce a social and cultural milieu for patients and staff which is more congruent with the norms of the larger society than like the norms of a special professional group.

Patient-Staff Socialization. Socialization of patients and staff into hospital systems is another area which is limitedly understood or may be unknown to health personnel, and yet it is important for health workers so that they can help people become acceptable members of the hospital without unduly losing their sociocultural and personal identity. Socialization is necessary for any patient's survival; as it provides guidelines for his behavior which is necessary if he is to obtain essential health services and move toward a recovery state. Whether we realize it or not, every patient goes through a process of socialization in which he learns the norms of the different professional groups and determines how his own norms fit with the professional ones. In the process of socialization he learns about the routines of hospital services, the differences between professional and nonprofessional services, the expectations of the staff, and the ways to get services in crisis and noncrisis situations. Socialization is as vital to patients as it is for new staff members entering a health system. To date, there is limited information about the various methods used by patients and staff for socialization, and about the consequences of these methods. It is perhaps, one of the most critical areas of study for the future.

Hospitals as a Replica of the Community. Another misconception about the hospital which is often heard is that "our hospital is a replica of the community at large." This assumption can often be challenged, for the hospital may or may not have similar features to the community in which it is located. In general, there is a recognition that hospitals exist in a community, but they may be antithetical to the social structure and culture of the larger community.

Commonly, health personnel perceive the hospital as a special community with its own unique social organization, cultural norms, and practices. Hospitals, as institutions, tend to develop their own normative and interpersonal styles of operation which may be quite foreign to people who live in the community in which the hospital is located. Anthropological studies have revealed the relationship of hospitals to the community in which they are located and have found varying kinds of relationships and structures. For example, Caudill's work revealed how the psychiatric hospital was a small community in itself and had special patterns of staff-patient interaction and cultural norms. Other social scientists have discovered that, in general, health institutions may have quite different structural and normative patterns from the communities they serve. From the author's consultation and practice experience in a number of hospitals in various communities, she can report that practically each hospital was like a subculture or little community of its own, and that it was necessary to learn about each hospital's cultural health and social norms. For example, in one community the author found six distinct kinds of hospital cultures, with each having its own norms, style of operation, and distinct social structure. There were only limited features reflecting the general cultural norms of the larger community. Hospital cultures are not only different from community cultures, but they differ among themselves.

Role-taking: Static and Dynamic Aspects. Finally, among the list of common conceptions and misconceptions about system behavior there exists the belief that, once an individual enters a hospital, he will be greatly limited in his personal and role freedom because he takes on the role of being a patient. Role-taking and the range of freedom for patients to take sick or well roles warrants systematic study to help us understand what happens to patients in a hospital or health agency. Social anthropologists tend to support the view that there is considerable freedom in most of the roles that any person or group takes. For example, in the role of mother a person has a wide latitutde of functions to perform, activities to engage in, and expectations to meet so that one does not need to feel unduly "cramped" by being a mother. If the role becomes restrictive or gives a person feelings of being severely limited, it is often due to the person's own perceptions and narrow expectation of the role. Moreover, when one takes a role such as that of the patient, one should not presume that the patient should be a victim of a role forever. Indeed, some roles are more changeable than others. For example, a mother or father role is generally more lasting over a span of time than a patient role. However, some staff members may try to keep patients in perpetual sick roles or the patient may be reluctant to relinquish his sick role.

Role might best be viewed as a structured sociographical position in relation to others and their expectations, and one which has both dynamic and static features to it. Every individual (patient and staff) takes a role, often by virtue of his own actions and reactions to the people around him, and he may emphasize certain aspects of his role and de-emphasize others. Essentially, the way the individual perceives, interprets, and acts in a role will largely determine the role-pattern response from others. There are, however, certain normative behavior expectations with which other people confront a person who occupies a culturally defined role. For example, the man who takes on a father role in American culture is expected to provide the basic income for his family and will legally and socially protect his family members. With some individuals, this role is narrowly perceived with only limited variations permitted. There is also the role expectation of the nurse, i.e., that she should be attentive, nurturant, and helpful to persons who are sick. The public expects that the nurse will be protective and supportive, and will provide for the physical and emotional needs of sick persons. The way the nurse views her role will influence how other people perceive her in her role. She should be aware of her own view of herself in a nurse role and she should also be sensitive to her patient's views of her in that role. Some patients may have more of a "fixed" view than others about the role of a nurse. Cultural groups sometimes may unconsciously or even overtly ask her to modify her nursing behavior to conform to their role expectations. For example, the patient may wish the nurse to assume an employers role. Accordingly, the nurse has opportunity to modify aspects of her role so that patients can see other features of it which can be therapeutic for him—and a role which he may not have thought would be helpful to him for his recovery. Role stereotypes about the nurse in our society exist and can limit the nurse's professional image and endeavors. For example, the nurse may be viewed as a person who gives *only* physical care to patients, or a person who never does anything without the physician's orders. Again, the nurse may be viewed as a servant to the physician. These stereotype images must be modified to show new and expanding roles and subroles of the professional nurse.

In a comparable manner, the patient may be perceived by health personnel to have a limited role, and this limitation may influence his recovery. Often patients are able to extend the nurse's and physician's perceptions and expectations of his patient role, and it is of interest to observe the way in which a patient can educate health personnel. There should be freedom for patients to show a variety of role (repertoire) behavior. They should have the freedom to respond to others in different ways in order to obtain certain kinds of services and in order to express their own behavioral tendencies. It is true that there are some static normative features related to being a patient, but there are also dynamic aspects too.

In some settings, the role of the patient may be rigidly perceived and defined, and so the patient has to behave in certain limited ways. For example, a patient may be expected always to cooperate with the staff in certain ways before he can be dismissed from the hospital. Sometimes, the patient chooses not be be cooperative, since it does not fit his personality and his patient role image, and so he struggles against the staff (sometimes at his own expense). Often when the range of role behavior and the opportunities for change are extremely limited, the patient literally goes along with the system in order to get out of the system. Role-taking has both static and dynamic attributes, and largely depends on one's perception and experience with role-taking and role stereotyping behavioral tendencies.

Although there are other misconceptions and conceptions about sociocultural systems, hopefully the above factors serve to identify some of the major ones. Now let us look briefly at the nurse's perceptions of sociocultural systems.

Nurses' Perceptions of Sociocultural Systems

Lately, nurses completing baccalaureate and graduate programs in nursing are becoming more knowledgeable about and interested in social system behavior. And nurses enrolled in doctoral programs in anthroupology and sociology are not only knowledgeable about system behavior, but several are actively involved in research studies related to system behavior. There is, however, a sizeable core of nurses who have limited awareness of how systems influence them and their patients. As one listens to nurses who have not had preparation about system behavior, one detects a struggle to understand the terms and concepts and their significance. Several nurses whom I have had in classes have said, "System behavior is a vague, diffuse and 'out there' idea which is hard to understand." Initially, several nurses thought that it is so intangible and vague that they prefer to leave the subject to social scientists. At the same time, there are some nurses eager to grasp social system ideas and to use them in patient care and staff relationships. There are also nurses, amazingly enough, who have gained, through their own self-study, fairly comprehensive understanding of system behavior and are eager for further insights about the subject. Some nurses are quite reluctant to become agents of change in system behavior. It is true that they can identify aspects of system behavior that need to be modified, but they are afraid to modify group behavior because "it seems so large and uncertain a task in a social system." Some of the reluctance may be related to the belief that system behavior should not be changed, or if it is changed it must be done by a group of experts. It is reasonable to predict that as nurses become more knowledgeable about system behavior, they will venture to make more modifications in it and, in doing so, can become effective collaborators with applied social scientists.

Some nurses tend to view social and cultural systems as barriers against giving high quality care to patients. The "system," to them, is like a huge "immovable obstacle" which is thwarting the nurse in helping her patients. With this image of systems, the nurse feels helpless and powerless to effect changes, and so she assumes a "hands off" position. Other nurses view social and cultural systems as malevolent forces which have limited positive features. They know hospitals can be dysfunctional, and yet no one knows what to do about it. Nurses viewing health institutions in this way need help in reexamining systems, so that they can gain new perceptions and discover ways to be a positive force in changing system behavior. Many of the nurses with whom the author has discussed system behavior were employed in large complex hospitals in which the bureaucratic features of the hospital were oppressive and well established and do pose problems in changing system ways.

In general, nurses' perceptions about social and cultural systems vary in proportion to the amount of educational preparation the nurse has had in understanding systems. Whether or not nurses take an active part in understanding system behavior and act as agents of system change will be largely dependent upon their knowledge and involvement in social system activities. One thing remains certain—that any nurse who is employed in a health institution will continue to be a part of system behavior. For system behavior is an inevitable phenomenon which is an integral dimension of our institutions, especially health institutions.

The Culture of the Hospital

Hospitals are fascinating, special, and complex cultural institutions in our society. As we have already mentioned, hospitals have their own special norms of behavior and patterns of interaction which make the hospital an institution of its own kind. Although some hospitals may have highly idiosyncratic rules of behavior with their own cultural norms, still one can also identify some common and generalized features of many hospitals in the United States. These general features, however, have not been rigorously examined in a wide sample of hospitals. Nonetheless, they are discussed in the literature and talked about in hospital settings. A few of these general features have been formulated by the author and will be noted here.

An individual entering the hospital soon discovers that the hospital is a highly complex institution which has the aim of giving health services to people through combined professional and business-oriented norms. The hospital is characterized as being comprised of a variety of health and business personnel who are expected to carry out defined and specialized services in relation to the patient and staff. The patient is expected to learn through direct participant observation and through various subtle communication media what his role is in the hospital and what the cultural norms of the hospital are. The patient must also learn which activities are performed by the various professional, nonprofessional, and other persons employed in the hospital system. Discovering who does what, when, and how is often a sizeable task for the patient and especially if he is critically ill.

Of most importance, the patient will discover that the cultural system of the hospital has status and power invested primarily in a certain professional group, namely, the physician group. Traditionally, and still so today, the physician is the person at the top of the organizational pyramid who has obvious power and prestige over the other professional groups in the hospital system. It is the physician who is perceived as the person who makes decisions about patient's welfare and treatment and who determines the time period the patient will spend in the hospital. More and more, efforts are being made to reduce the centralized power invested in physicians so that authority, decision-making, status, and prestige are distributed in an equitable way to other professional groups according to their professional abilities and preparation. With current efforts to decentralize power and authority in some progressive hospitals, nurses and other professional groups are being recognized for their independent decisions, responsibilities and professional skills. This trend, long overdue, should yield better and quicker services to patients, especially when various rights and privileges are institutionally sanctioned as belonging to different professional groups.

Since *health care is primarily a function of the nursing profession*, the cultural rules governing health care are gradually changing to give more legitimate power and authority to nurses in order that they may have more freedom and autonomy in the decision making involved in nursing care. The nurse is becoming aware of the role of power status and authority in an institution and how it can influence the quality of care to patients. Nonetheless, the concepts of power and authority and their consequences for staff and patients are still a relatively new area of concern for many nurses. All too frequently, there are major conflicts and stresses in hospitals related to power use and abuse, and a variety of conflicts related to the proper use of lines of authority. The works of King,[9] Smith,[10] Wooden,[11] Caudill,[12] Etzioni,[13] and others can help the nurse understand some of the common conflicts and stresses related to power, authority, and status in social structure of a hospital.

The hospital subculture in the United States is largely a world of sickness where staff members hustle around to observe, treat, and care for strangers. To date, there are no full ethnographic studies of how people actually become patients and respond to the large and baffling world of sickness which characterizes the hospital. King has identified the hospital subculture as one which: "1) lacks privacy, 2) has strange equipments and language, 3) has unusual sights, sounds and smells, and 4) has unvarying routines."[14] In addition, the hospital subculture has both implicit and explicit rules about what behavior is acceptable or nonacceptable. Cultural rules govern the patient's behavior as well as that of his family and friends. One of the implicit rules of behavior is that the patient must show a desire to move from the sick role to a well role and then to stay well. This norm of behavior is revealed to the patient in many ways. If patients show signs of behavior contrary to this norm, the staff may subtly reject the patient, avoid him, or give him an early release from the hospital under the aegis of various kinds of rationalized staff explanations. A patient who has suicidal tendencies or shows malingering behavior is generally viewed as a deviant—one who does not follow the expected norms of patient behavior. These patients are viewed as "problem patients," since they challenge the staff to understand their behavior.

Another implicit cultural norm found in a hospital is that *patients should acquiesce to the authority, directives, and help of professional staff, and particularly of the physician*. Hospital personnel use a variety of techniques and methods to place patients in a subordinate position. The implicit assumption is that the staff has the knowledge, skills, and ability to help the patient only if the patient will acquiesce to and cooperate. The shift for some patients, who in their daily life have been in a superordinate, command, or control position toward others, and are now in the opposite role of depending upon the thinking, decisions, and actions of others, can be a source of great stress and conflict. Patients who try to maintain a superordinate position in respect to the professional staff are in a vulnerable and awkward position for receiving help, and they may be rejected, avoided, or given minimal attention.

Patients are expected to learn that *the cultural norm of adapting to a variety of hospital routiens, rules, treatment modalities, and staff expectations is necessary in order to successfully get in and out of the hospital.* It is hard to perceive from the patient's viewpoint the kinds of stresses and anxieties he encounters as he adjusts to hospital rituals, treatment practices, and other expectations. Considerable physical, psychological, and social energy must be exerted to cope with this cultural norm expectation. For the patient to manage reasonably to predict what may happen to him daily, hourly, weekly, and monthly while in the hospital, involves considerable cognitive efforts and psychological involvement. Furthermore, if the patient fails to adjust to the expectations of the hospital staff, he usually encounters new problems such as difficulty in getting his medications on time, insufficient information to know where to go for special treatments, and lack of concern for his special personal needs or comforts.

Social and cultural adjustments and expectations of others are a normal part of life and of most hospital cultures. In addition, the patient has physical and psychological adaptations to make which may be related to the loss of limb or an organ. During an illness experience, the patient may need to adapt to strange new diets, refrain from seeing his family, secure proper bed rest, and so on, all depending upon his particular health problem. Nurses often witness first-hand the patient's efforts to adjust to special health problems such as facial disfigurement, extensive body mutilation, a permanent disability, or the death of a loved one. Accompanying these expected adaptations, the patient has to also adjust to the different cultural backgrounds of the staff. Patients who have never been cared for by an Afro-American nurse or a Jewish-American physician, for example, may have to adjust to special cultural roles besides those of the hospital. Consideration of these adjustments and others relative to the hospital environment should help the reader become aware of the many factors the patient needs to adjust to as part of the general cultural norms of most hospitals today.

In the subculture of the hospital, there are also *certain modes of communication that are expressed by verbal, nonverbal, and technological means* and there are *rules* which govern communication between patients and staff. Determining the specific modes and rules of communication used in a particular hospital between the staff members and between the staff and patients is a fascinating study in itself. There are discernible rules of communication in any hospital, but the patterns usually vary depending upon the size of the hospital, its traditional communication modes, the physical structure of the hospital, and other factors. In general, communication pathways in most hospitals tend to be complex and covert and the patient has to determine the essential communication pathways to get his needs met. There are, in general, both formal and informal communication patterns in the hospital which are governed by certain rules of sending and receiving messages between the staff and patients. The patient generally relies on other patients and the nurse to help him find out the various rules and pathways of communication. Frequently, the patient may have only partial information and a few rules available to him about the modes and pathways of the hospital communication system. Such partial information may seriously handicap the patient in receiving help when he needs it most.

Finally, *the hospital subculture expects that patients will accept the physical, psychological, sociological, and cultural environment of a hospital.* The sick world environment, with its wide variety of human illnesses and a different kind of physical environment from one's home, is part of the hospital culture. Living with two or more sick persons in your immediate environment and over a period of time may be difficult for some patients. Hearing, seeing, and talking with sick people for many hours, days, or weeks are realities of the hospital subculture. And finally, there is the total cultural environment of the hospital, with its constant movement of people and strange objects to some place for something. The movement of people and objects may be exceedingly baffling and anxiety-producing to some who are in the hospital for the first time.

It is recognized that more research is needed to study the specific nature of each hospital culture as well as the general or any universal features of many hospitals. Both positive and negative effects can be identified with people who experience the hospital subculture. Although it is hard today in our society to conceive of helping patients without a hospital, still there are possibilities that a hospital is not the only means of administering health needs of people. The challenge to find new ways of helping people which will ease the adjustment and socialization process remains virtually unexplored. At the same time, it is recognized in our society that hospitals are necessary institutions which tend to increase in number and size. Moreover, the hospital would probably not have grown to be the large industry it has in our culture, had it not been that it does serve some important and expected functions and needs. What will be the culture of hospitals in the future? Will there be a change in the norms of the hospital and its social system? What innovations will maximize the eufunctions of the hospital and minimize its dysfunctions? These and other questions await serious thought and systematic research by our health professionals and social scientists.

In this chapter, the focus has been on health institutions as social and cultural institutions. Several definitions and fundamental explanations regarding social and cultural systems have been presented. Hopefully, this chapter has provided some key concepts and definitions about system behavior so that the nurse who has limited knowledge about system behavior can begin to work within systems in an informed way. The next decade will challenge nurses to become more knowledgeable about system behavior and will make explicit their role in changing and maintaining effective health care nursing systems.

FOOTNOTES

[1] *Webster's New International Dictionary.* Third Edition, 1968.

[2] William Caudill, and others, "Social Structure and Interaction Process on a Psychiatric Ward," *American Journal of Orthopsychiatry,* Vol. 22, April 1952, pp. 314-334.

[3] John Cummings and Elaine Cummings, "Mental Health Education in a Canadian Community," in Benjamin D. Paul, Ed., *Health, Culture, and Community,* New York: Russell Sage Foundation, 1955, pp. 43-69.

[4] Alfred Stanton and Morris S. Schwartz, *The Mental Hospital,* New York: Basic Books, Inc., 1954.

[5] Erving Goffman, "On the Characteristics of Total Institutions," *Asylums:* 10,10,12;Essays in the Social Situation of Mental Patients and Other Inmates, Garden City, New York: Doubleday Anchor, 1961, pp.1-124.

[6] Otto von Mering and Stanley H. King, *Remotivating the Mental Patient,* New York: Russell Sage Foundation, 1957.

[7] William Caudill, *The Psychiatric Hospital as a Small Society,* Cambridge, Massachusetts: Harvard University Press, 1958.

[8] Laurence J. Peter and Raymond Hull, *The Peter Principle,* New York: Bantam Book Edition, 1970.

[9] Stanley H. King, *Perceptions of Illness and Medical Practice,* New York: Russell Sage Foundation, 1962.

[10] Harvey Smith, "The Sociological Study of Hospitals," unpublished doctoral dissertation, University of Chicago, Chicago, 1949.

[11] Howard E. Wooden, "The Hospital's Purpose is the Patient, But—," *Modern Hospital,* Vol. 92, January 1959, pp. 90-96.

[12] William Caudill, *op. cit.* pp. 314-334.

[13] Amitai Etzioni, "Authority Structure and Organization Effectiveness," *Administrative Science Quarterly,* Vol. 4, June 1959, 44-67.

[14] Stanley King, *op. cit.,* pp. 350-358.

SUGGESTED REFERENCES

Emily Mumford and J. K. Skipper, Jr., *Sociology in Hospital Care,* New York: Harper and Row, 1967.

Jeannette Folta and Edith Deck, *A Sociological Framework for Patient Care,* New York: John Wiley and Sons, 1966.

Stanley H. King, "The Hospital: An Analysis in Terms of Social Structure," *Perceptions of Illness and Medical Practice,* New York: Russell Sage Foundation, 1962, pp. 307-348.

Temple Burling et al, *The Give and Take in Hospitals: A Study in Human Organization in Hospitals,* New York: Putnam, 1956, pp. 81-160.

Talcott Parsons, "Some Definitions of Health and Illness in the Light of American Values and Social Structure," *Social Structure and Personality.* New York: Free Press of Glencoe, 1964.

11 Ethnoscience: A Promising Research Approach to Improve Nursing Practice[1]

The relationship between the field of nursing and the field of anthropology is still largely unknown and unexplored. Once this relationship is established, it is reasonable to predict that a wealth of new insights and a deepened appreciation of man's behavior and development will be forthcoming. Since anthropology is committed to the scientific study of man in our immediate American environment and in the most remote places in the world, this field has much to contribute to nursing. Most important, both the fields of anthropology and nursing are concerned with man's health and illness behavior; this is the initial common bond which brings the two fields close together. Nursing needs anthropology's broad knowledge and special insights into man's behavior now and in a depth-time perspective. Anthropology needs the rich descriptive knowledge from the field of nursing about man's behavior under acute and chronic threats to his health status. In this chapter, an anthropological research method is discussed to stimulate nurses' thinking about a fresh and new research approach to the study of health-illness systems of behavior of people with different cultural and subcultural backgrounds.

The Patient's View of Illness is Important

One of the new and most challenging problems for researchers in health and social sciences is to accurately describe and explain man's health and illness behavior *from the patient's viewpoint.* In the past, patient behavior has been described largely from different professional group members' perspectives and from "imposed" inferences from the patient. The recent interest in and emphasis on the importance of discovering the patient's view of his illness is opening new challenges to health personnel. It challenges us to understand more fully how the patient knows and understands his illness, how he desires to be helped, and the ways health personnel can help him. Most important, it provides an accurate basis on which health personnel can get to know and help the patient. This approach recognizes that patients are capable of telling us about their illness, about the way their illness has affected them, and about the factors influencing the illness. Unfortunately, there are only a few places where health personnel give careful and full consideration to *the patient's view of his illness.*

Anthropologists have long stressed the importance of using information from the people they study and from first-hand informants in understanding a cultural group, its world view, and its way of living. Anthropologists also recognize that man tends to respond in a highly artificial way when placed in controlled or artifically-contrived settings, in contrast to the spontaneous and natural responses found in his familiar life settings. There is a need for rigorous scientific methods to study man's behavior in his natural environment, and especially for comparative studies of man in diverse cultural, social, and ecological settings. One of the most promising research approaches to the study of man in his natural environments, and from a comparative perspective, is the ethnoscience research method. It is a relatively new approach in anthropology and is being referred to as the "new ethnography" of the discipline. It is more of a sophisticated and rigorous field study method than the old ethnographic approach and has a rapidly growing body of enthusiastic supporters who believe in its merits and its future scientific potentialities.

Ethnoscience: Definition and Goals

Ethnoscience refers to the systematic study of the way of life of a designated cultural group with the purpose of obtaining an accurate account of the people's behavior and how they perceive and interpret their universe. Based upon the principle that a people *can* and *do* classify ideas and experiences in their universe, ethnoscience is a careful and conscientious systemization of a cultural group's cognitions. The aim of ethnoscience is to reduce the chaos of data about a cultural group by classifying such information so that it accurately portrays the *indigenous people's views* to others, and offers support for the validity and reliability of ethnographic data. The ethnoscientist's task is to study and classify data about a cultural group so that it is meaningful both to the people being studied and to strangers trying to understand the culture. Frake states that ethnoscience concentrates on "discerning how people construe their world experience from the way they talk about it."[2] *The ultimate goal of ethnoscience is to discover the culturally relevant cognitive system of the bearers of a culture.* From classified data, the ethnographer (or scientist) obtains data which has a high degree of validity and reliability to the local people and by the scientific analysis of components of a culture. From this basic knowledge, the scientist constructs meaningful hypotheses and theoretical positions which can then be tested. The ethnoscientific approach is valued because it provides rich data for the specification, generalization, and prediction of human behavior.

The idea of eliciting and studying *a cultural group's own perceptions of and knowledge about their world* is not a new endeavor in the field of anthropology. Early ethnographers recognized that in obtaining data from a group whose cultural background was different from their own, they needed to obtain the native's point of view. Malinowski, a social anthropologist, stated in 1922 that "the final goal, of which an Ethnographer should never lose sight ... is, briefly, to grasp the native's point of view, his relation to life, to realise *his* vision and *his* world."[3] What is new is the rigorous method of systematic data classification according to new ethnographic and linguistic methods, and the use of scientific principles to provide an accurate collection of and analysis of data. Before identifying some of the principles related to the general ethnoscience method, I shall pause to briefly consider the above statements about ethnoscience aims and methods in relation to the health science field, and especially to nursing.

If the ethnoscience approach were used by health personnel, it would provide an "inside view" and hopefully valid data about the patient, his family, and the significant people in his community who directly or indirectly influence the patient's behavior. The ethnoscience approach would help the nurse conscientiously obtain the patient's views about his health and illness behavior, and then classify these data into units of behavior in a systematic way. The nurse would discover aspects of the patient's behavior that she ordinarily would not obtain by her usual methods of eliciting information about a patient. The method would be essentially a new approach for health personnel who traditionally tend to use their own cultural and professional cognitions about a patient's behavior and assume they accurately reflect the patient's views and behavior. It seems long overdue that in order to provide meaningful and effective health services to patients, systematic focus must be given to the patient's personal and cultural views regarding health and illness.

Currently, there are big gaps between the professional person's and the patient's perceptions and experiences related to health and illness. Perceptual and cognitive difference can give rise to serious difficulties in communicating with patients and in establishing therapeutic relationships with them. I refer to these gaps as "cultural discrepancies in health norms." Sometimes these norm discrepancies become so conceptually noticeable that patients find it difficult to understand their illness and the behavior of health personnel who are caring for them. To resolve this dilemma, patients may silently and graciously refuse to return for health care because they do not understand how these services are helping them.

People who come from varying cultural backgrounds bring with them their own health practices and beliefs about what they think can help them. How often have professional staff neglected to explore the patient's perceptions and cognitions of illness? Anthropological studies reveal that patients and their families often abandon temporarily their own indigenous health practices in order to satisfy the expectations of professional workers. Furthermore, these patients frequently return to their traditional practices when they are away from professional people. Studies also reveal the tendency of professional workers to view indigenous health practices as nonscientific, superstitious, and ridden with magic. But in studying indigenous health systems, scientists have discovered many positive, therapeutic, and scientific features about folk health beliefs and practices.[4,5] The ethnoscience method can help professional people systematically study and order data relating to particular cultures. The ethnoscience method provides for some exciting and challenging new breakthroughs in nursing and medical research. The recent interest in studying health and illness from an indigenous point of view gives promise not only of a more valid basis for health practices, but also a broader understanding of health practices of people in their natural living environments. Let us turn to further aspects about the ethnoscience approach, especially its basic assumptions, principles and theoretical views.

Assumptions, Principles and Theoretical Views of Ethnoscience

One of the basic assumptions of ethnoscience is that a cultural group perceives and orders its universe in a patterned, orderly, and identifiable way. The ordering of people's cognitions in a knowledgeable way is not only characteristic of *homo sapiens*, but tends to be a necessary requirement for man's cultural, social, physiological and psychological survival. It is, therefore, the scientist's task to discover the way man orders and knows his universe and to search for the rules which support this method of ordering.

With the ethnoscience method, there are two important concepts—

"emic" and "etic"—which help us understand and refine data. The *emic approach* has been succinctly defined by French as the means which sets out "to discover and describe the behavioral system (of a given culture) in its own terms, identifying not only the structural cognitive units of the people but also the structural classes to which they belong."[6] Anthropological research has revealed, for instance, that color is perceived and classified differently by different cultures. Some cultures have only four color classes such as red, yellow, blue and green; whereas, another culture has seven definite structural classes of color. Moreover, different principles for classifying such data are used by different cultures, and so the scientist must discover the local perceptual and cognitive structure of color classification. In brief, *emic* analysis is concerned with the way members of a local culture order and interpret their world. In contrast, the *etic approach* concentrates on features which may belong to more than one culture, or to the sum of all the significant attributes of folk classifications which can be found among a number of cultures. In the *etic approach*, folk classifications may have relevance beyond one particular indigenous group. In fact, a local classification may have some universal features which help in the ultimate quest for broad domains of verified knowledge about man. Sturtevant states that a culture generally has shared classifications with other cultures; however, one must not assume that every etic difference is necessarily *emic*.[7] Generally, different emic systems are locally analyzed with the specific culture in mind and these emic units may or may not be found in the etic analysis.

Since any two cultures tend to differ in the way they classify experience, the ethnoscientist has to look for a potential range of different categories and sets of categories relating to a particular phenomenon. Thus another important ethnoscience principle is that one must *determine the boundaries of the major categories* being analyzed by taking clues from the local indigenous people. For example, anthropologists recognize that "aunt" is not a universal category in studying kinship systems, even though it is found in our Anglo-American kinship system. In other cultures, there may be different sets of "aunt-like" categories. Prior assumptions of researchers about the universality of categories and their domains may vary, and these variabilities must be recognized and identified. Knowledge about different kinds of subject matter categories and about category boundaries also provides important clues about the nature of relationship behavior in a culture. For example, a mother's brother is expected to offer protection and to give gifts to his nephew in many South African cultures by virtue of being classified "Mother's brother."

Another important principle in ethnoscience method is that *native linguistic labels of different categories have meaning and must be identified and described*. Knowledge of the local language and its linguistic structure is, of course, necessary for an accurate identification of the specific categories and their attributes. The labels of the different classificatory categories are called *lexemes,* a term which refers to a "meaningful form whose signification cannot be inferred from a knowledge of anything else in the languge."[8]

Closely allied to the identification and meaning of terms, the ethnoscience researchers must study *contrasting sets of mutually exclusive segregates* which are generally found in the same cultural setting. *Segregates are composed of attributes which distinguish sets of items from one another.* As Conklin and Frake say, these segregates "share exclusively in at least one defining feature . . . i.e., that which characterizes the setting in which they are found."[9, 10] Essentially, the idea is to look for mutually exclusive attributes of an item and contrasting sets of data that are distinguishable from one another. The contrasts, too, have rules governing their existence and meaning. For example, segregates for sick and well behavior may exist and serve as two contrasting sets of data which can be distinguishable between one another. Another example, is that there may be two contrasting sets of data about a hamburger which clearly identifies two "kinds" of hamburgers in our society. It is important for the researcher to identify the contrastive features and meaning of these sets of data. The term, *paradigm,* is also used, and refers to a *set of segregates which can be distinguished by their meaning, i.e.,* a set which shares some features that are not shared by other segregates in the same set.[11, 12] Only two segregates can be viewed as a paradigm; however, there may be more than two sub-sets. Since ethnoscientific work requires that the analysis reflect the cognitive system of the bearers of a culture and the rules for their classification of data, a componential analysis of a paradigm is performed in order to define these dimensions of contrasts and the attributes which characterize the segregates in a set. Componential analysis generally reflects those classificatory principles of the people being studied which are *"cognitively salient"* (*i.e.,* a psychological reality) to them.[13] However, the analysis may also reflect more of *"structural reality,"* or what Lounsbury calls "formal account."[14]

One of the last but most important principles of the ethnoscience method is to *identify the folk taxonomy* (the "emic" approach) by determining how the different segregates and contrasting sets are related to each other within their culture and within the hierarchial order of the sets. This requires a full critical study of the data collected in order to discover the critical attributes of a local folk taxonomy.

Application of the Method: Gadsup Health Practitioner Roles

Having briefly discussed the ethnoscientific approach, now we will consider an example which will enable us to understand the method better. Most of the groundbreaking applications of the ethnoscience method have been made in relation to kinship, to color, and to biological plant analyses. Only one ethnoscientific study of folk health classifications has been reported, namely, Metzger and Williams' investigation of the Tzeltal people.[15] In order to illustrate the ethnoscientific approach, the author will draw upon her own work with the health practitioner roles of the Gadsup people of the Eastern Highlands of New Guinea. The author has also used the ethnoscience method in studying a Spanish-speaking urban community group in a metropolitan city in the United States; however, this work is not yet complete.[16] The author recognizes that the method of studying health roles is new, and that the details of the method will need further refinement.

The table below reveals the ethnoscience world of the Gadsup health practitioner roles. The terms, categories, sub-sets, and segregates were derived by using the ethnoscientific method.

From the table on page 174, some fascinating deductions about the Gadsup health practitioner rules can be made from the three major segregates. In Segregate 1, *Village Male Curers and Preventionists*, one discovers that: (1) the males are primarily curers and preventionists, (2) males deal with crises and unnatural cases of illness, (3) males only treat adult males, and (4) males are the only villagers capable of curing supernatural forces, nature spirits, sorcery, and war illnesses. In Segregate 2, *Village Female Curers, Carers, and Preventionists*, one finds that: (1) females deal with care, cure, and prevention, (2) females work primarily as cure, care, and prevention agents for women, children, and small pigs, (3) no adult males are ever cared for directly by women, since women are potentials for the dreaded menstrual illness, (4) females work with daily and common village illnesses, (5) females are never expected to cure illnesses listed under Subset C of the Village Male Curers, and (6) women are the only persons knowledgeable about and skilled in childbirth practices (males must never intrude into this domain of knowledge and skill). In Segregate 3, *Non-Village Male Curers*, one finds the following features: (1) these men are perceived as curers and specialists, (2) there are two major categories, namely, the Gadsup non-villager and the European doctor-boys, (3) these specialists deal with inter-village, stranger-produced, and highly unknown (to the villagers) illnesses, (4) the specialists deal with illnesses which the village curers have not been able to cure, (5) specialists are given some form of recompense, either gifts, money, or services for their services, and (6) the specialists deal primarily with males and children, and only occasionally with adult females.

Implications for Nursing Care. The implications for nursing care and treatment can be readily identified from the above findings. Any professional nurse going into the Gadsup culture would have to identify her role under

TABLE I

ETHNOSCIENCE CATEGORIES OF GADSUP HEALTH PRACTITIONER ROLES

Paradigm → Gadsup Curers, Carers, and Preventionists (General Category)

Segregates		
1. Village Male Curers and Preventionists (Generalists)*	2. Village Female Curers, Carers, & Preventionists (Generalists)*	3. Non-Village Male Curers (Specialists)*

Paradigm and Subsets		

A. *War Curers*
  1. Fighting curers
  2. Arrow curers
B. *Sorcery Curers*
  1. Intravillage sorcery
  2. Intervillage sorcery
C. *Taboo Curers*
  1. War taboos
  2. Food taboos
  3. Breaking culture taboos
  4. Menstrual taboos
D. *Supernatural Curers*
E. *Nature Spirit Curers*
	A. *Childbirth Carers* (semi-specialists)
	B. *Women-Children Curers*
	  1. Children illnesses (both male & female)
	  2. Women illnesses
	  3. Small pig illnesses
	C. *Prevention of Village Illnesses*
	  1. Sorcery
	  2. Food taboos
	  3. Menstrual taboos
	  4. Garden taboos
	  5. General village taboos
	D. *Indirect Carers of Sick Men* (except for menstrual illnesses)
		A. *Gadsup Non-Village Curers*
		  1. War curers for "big-man" fighting illnesses
		  2. Sorcery curers for intervillage "death" sorcerers
		  3. Menstrual taboo illnesses of men
		  4. Illnesses caused by non-Gadsup strangers
		  5. Broken bone curers
		  6. Rare and unknown illnesses
		B. *European Doctor-Boys*
		  1. Pill-givers
		  2. Shot-givers
		  3. Child-checkers
		  4. Cut-openers at Kaiantu

*Prevention is an integral part of the curer's role.	*Curing is the primary focus in the curer's role.	*Cure, care, and prevention are integral parts of the curer's role.

Segregate 2 if she were to achieve successful and effective work with these people. If she wanted to serve as an agent of change, she would need to be keenly aware of all three segregates and subsets, she would need to work with practitioners on the basis of their traditional roles, and she would have to determine where role modification was feasible. To date, we have no systematic analysis of our own American cultural and subcultural group's health practitioner's roles. Instead, there are only generalized and vague descriptions of our various health practitioner roles as seen from the people's viewpoint.

In comparing the ethnohealth system of the Gadsup people with whatever health system you are accustomed to you will look for how health systems differ with respect to different categories and sub-categories of illnesses as people perceive and interpret their health-illness universe. Hopefully, this ethnoscience approach to the study of health systems will continue to be used so that a systematic identification of major patterns of ethnohealth systems of different cultures and subculture groups will be established. In a number of health systems, one could begin to identify *emic* and *etic* dimensions. But most important, the ethnoscience approach and findings from the research method should provide more valid and reliable data than is currently available. Our knowledge is meager about the health-illness cognitions of our patients and there is a great need for more precise knowledge if we are to achieve a more scientific and humanistic mode of care for different patient groups in the United States and elsewhere.

Merits of the Ethnoscience Method

In summary, there are a number of potential benefits that the ethnoscience method has to offer the cultural anthropologist and the nurse. First, the ethnoscience method should give us an accurate and fairly reliable picture of a cultural group or a patient's cognitions and perceptions of health and illness. Second, and most important, it emphasizes the benefits of looking through the patient's own eyes, ears, and experiences to develop an effective nursing care plan and approach. It offers valuable data upon which we can tailor-make and creatively build a nursing care plan—a plan in which the patient's world is given full consideration. Third, such data from a given health system and from a number of health systems will provide us with a sound basis for prediction studies and generalization hypotheses about sick and well behavior. Fourth, the findings from the ethnoscience method could help generate nursing theories on health and illness behavior which could be tested locally with a patient from a particular culture, or could be used to test etic hypotheses of universal health-illness systems. Fifth, accurately obtained ethnoscience data should considerably reduce guess work about patient's needs and behavior and, consequently, about treatment-care strategies. The ethnoscience approach should greatly reduce the tendency of medical personnel to unduly superimpose their health norms upon patients whose values and cultural norms are different from their own. As we discussed in Chapters 4 and 7, sometimes differences in professional and indigenous norms vary so markedly that it is confusing and stressful to patients. And lastly, the ethnoscience method of studying health-illness systems should give us a deeper appreciation for foreign cultures and foreign health systems. Using ethnoscience data, nurses could develop role-taking skill for any given ethnohealth system.

The ethnoscience method has the potential of increasing the reliability and validity of data on cognitive health-illness behavior. It offers us a new research approach to understanding the patient's health world so that we as professional health practitioners can be effective, constructive, and helpful. The discovery of new knowledge and the unfolding of new orders of knowledge is a rewarding experience for the research nurse who uses the ethnoscience approach. There are a growing number of nurse researchers who are earnestly seeking to improve the quality of care to patients; hopefully, the ethnoscience method will be of assistance to them. The ethnoscience approach is extremely relevant in the future goal of developing cross-cultural nursing practices and studying health systems of different cultural and subcultural groups in the world.

FOOTNOTES

[1] A version of this chapter was presented at the University of Iowa in October, 1968 under the sponsorship of Gamma Chapter of Sigma Theta Tau, the College of Nursing, and the Graduate School of the University of Iowa.

[2] Charles O. Frake, "The Ethnographic Study of Cognitive Systems," in T. Gladwin and W. C. Sturtevant (Eds.), *Anthropology and Human Behavior*, Washington: Anthropological Society of Washington, 1962, pp. 72-85.

[3] Bronislaw Malinowski, *Argonauts of the Western Pacific*, London: George Routledge & Sons, Ltd., 1922.

[4] Benjamin Paul (Ed.), *Health, Culture and Community*, New York: Russell Sage Foundation, 1955.

[5] Ari Kiev (Ed.), *Magic, Faith, and Healing*, London: The Free Press of Glencoe, Collier-Macmillan Ltd., 1964.

[6] David French, "The Relationship of Anthropology to Studies in Perception and Cognition," in S. Koch (Ed.), *Psychology: A Study of a Science*, New York: McGraw-Hill, 6, pp. 388-428.

[7] William Sturtevant, "Studies in Ethnoscience," *American Anthropologist*, Special Publication on Transcultural Cognitions, A. Kimball Romney and Roy Goodwin D'Andrade, Part 2, 66(3), 1964, pp. 99-131.

[8]Harold C. Conklin, "Lexicographical Treatment of Folk Taxonomies," *International Journal of American Linguistics*, 28: 2, Part 4, 1962a, pp. 119-141.
[9]Harold C. Conklin, *Ibid*. 28:2, Part 4, 1962a.
[10]Charles O. Frake, "The Ethnographic Study of Cognitive Systems," in T. Gladwin and W. G. Sturtevant (Eds.), *Anthropology and Human Behavior*, Washington: Anthropological Society of Washington, 1962, pp. 72-85.
[11]Harold C. Conklin, *Ibid*, 28:2, Part 4, 1962a, pp. 119-141.
[12]Ward H. Goodenough, "Componential Analysis and the Study of Meaning," *Language*, 32(2), 1956a, pp. 195-216.
[13]Floyd G. Lounsbury, "A Formal Account of the Crow and Omaha-Type Kinship Terminologies," in W. H. Goodenough (Ed.), *Explorations in Cultural Anthropology: Essays Presented to George Peter Murdock*, New York: McGrawHill, 1964.
[14]Floyd G. Lounsbury, *Ibid*.
[15]Duane Metzger and Gerald Williams, "Tenejapa Medicine I: The Curer," *Southwestern Journal of Anthropology*, 19(2), 1963a, pp. 216-34.
[16]Madeleine Leininger, *Field Study Observations with Spanish-Speaking Peoples in an Urban Communicy, 1966-69*, unpublished report, 1969.

SUGGESTED REFERENCES

Gerald Berreman, "Anemic and Emetic Analysis in Social Anthropology," *American Anthropologist*, 1966, 68:346-354.
Robbins Burling, "Cognition and Componential Analysis: God's Truth or Hocuspocus?" *American Anthropologist*, 1964, 66:20-28; 120-122.
H. C. Conklin, "Hanunoo Color Categories," *Southwestern Journal of Anthropology*, 1955, 11:339-344.
Charles Frake, "The Ethnographic Study of Cognitive Systems," in *Anthropology and Human Behavior*, ed. T. Gladwin and W. G. Sturtevant, Washington: Anthropological Society of Washington, 1962, pp. 72-85. Reproduced by permission of the Anthropological Society of Washington.
T. Gladwin and W. G. Sturtevant, Introduction to paper by Frake, *Anthropology and Human Behavior*, Washington: Anthropological Society of Washington, 1962, pp. 72-73.
Ward Goodenough, "Componential Analysis and the Study of Meaning," *Language*, 1956, 32:195-216.
Pertti J. Pelto, *Anthropological Research: The Structure of Inquiry*, New York: Harper and Row, 1970, pp. 67-87.

Kenneth Pike, *Language in Relation to a Unified Theory of the Structure of Human Behavior,* Vol. 1, Glendale, Calif: Summer Institute of Linguistics, 1954.

William G. Sturtevant, "Studies in Ethnoscience," *American Anthropologist, 1964,66 (part 2):99-131.*

A. F. C. Wallace and John W. Atkins, "The Meaning of Kinship Terms," *American Anthropologist,* 1960, 62:58-80.

Index

Anthropology, as a unifying science, 7
  basic and applied, 14
  contributions of, 18-24
  cultural, 11-12
  definition of, 4
  ideal goal of, 9
  linguistic, 14
  methods of, 9
  of nursing, goal of, 18
  physical, 10
  psychological, 13-14
  social, 12-13
  sociology and differences between, 12
  subfields of, 9-14
  See Child rearing, Cross-cultural comparative perspective, Culture concept, Health-illness behavior, Holistic and cultural approach, Longitudinal perspective of man, Participant observation field-study methd, Socialization processes.
Archaeology, 11
Argyris, C., 79

Beeker, Howard S., 24
Behavior, formal system, 147
  informal system, 147
Bennett, Leland R., 61
Birdwhistell, Ray L., 26, 39
Bohannon, Paul, 35
Brown, Esther Lucille, 39

Case studies,
  Afro-American, 94-96, 104-106
  Cheyenne and Anglo-American couple, 107-110
  Czech-American, 101-103
  German-American, 86-90
  Italian-American, 90-91
  Mexican-American, 103-104
  Spanish-speaking, 91-94

Case Studies *(Continued)*
  Swedish-American, 106-107
  Vietnamese child, 128-144
Caudill, William, 39, 149, 157, 162
Child-rearing, 22-23, 128-144
Community field-study method, 2, 6
Conklin, H. C., 172
Cross-cultural and comparative perspective, 19
Cultural context of behavior, definition of, 111
  learning, 112
  Spanish-American, 111-126
  See also Case studies
Culturally-tailored nursing care plans, 21, 85, 99
Culture concept, 20
Culture, definition of, 48
Cultural shock, definition of, 48
Cultural system, definition of, 147
Cultural values, changing a patient's, 100
  definition of, 51
  optimum health as a, 52
Cummings, John and Elaine, 149

DeLaguna, Frederica, 6

Emic approach, 171
Ethnocentrism, and non-Western health norms, 46
  definition of, 19
Ethnography, 12
Ethnolinguistics, 14
Ethnoscience, assumptions, principles, theoretical views of, 170-172
  definition and goals of, 168-170
  of the Gadsup health practitioner roles, 174
  merits of, 175
  research method of, 168
Etic approach, 171
Etzioni, Amitai, 162
Folk-practitioners, Spanish-American, 120-121
Frake, Charles, 169, 172

179

Geer, Blanche, 24
Goffman, Irving, 149

Hallowell, Irving, 35
Hanson, Robert C., 123
Health-illness behavior, 4, 22
  cultural discrepancies in, 170
  patients view of, 168
  self-care adaptations, 32
  See also Case studies
Herskovits, Melville J., 7, 48
Holistic and cultural approach, 1, 21-22

Ideal culture, 50

Kimball, Solon, 39
Kinesics, 26
King, Stanley H., 149, 162

Language, culture, personality and race, relationship to, 26
  non-, symbols, 26
  See also Case studies
Linguistics, comparative historical, 14
  descriptive, 14
Linkage concept, 123
Longitudinal perspective of man, 5, 18

Malinowski, Bronislaw, 35
Manifest culture, 50
Material culture, 6, 49
McCabe, Garcia S., 39
Mead, Margaret, 39, 45

Non-material culture, 6, 49
Nurse-client relationship, 30-31, 156-157
  See also Case studies
Nursing, apprenticeship method in traditional culture of, 72-73
  as a profession today, 69
  definition of, 31
  education in new culture of, 65
  education in traditional culture of, 65
  function of, 162
  instrumental role behavior in new culture of, 77
  1937 Curriculum Guide and standardization of, 74
  views of, 29

Nursing *(Continued)*
  views of nurse in traditional culture of, 68, 76-77
  views of self in new culture of, 80
  views of self in traditional culture of, 65, 67

Participant observation field-study method, 24, 64
Pearsall, Marion, 24
Populations, genetic variations in, 10

Reisman, David, 65
Role, definition of, 158
  patient expectations of, 100
  relinquishing of, 153
  taking of, 153
  See also Case studies

Saunders, Lyle, 39, 123
Schwartz, Morris S., 149
Self-other awareness, 35
Smith, Harvey, 162
Social, groups, 8
  institutions, 8
  structures, 12
  systems, 146
Socialization process, 22-23
  in case study, 86-90
  patient-staff, 156-157
Sociocultural systems, components of, 152-153
Stanton, Alfred, 149
Sturtevant, William S., 171
Subculture, definition of, 51
  of nursing, 64
Subsystem, social and cultural dimensions of, 149-151
System, as barrier, 60
  closed, definition of, 148
  cultural, 147
  dysfunctions of, 155
  eufunctions of, 155
  health institution as a cultural and social, 145-165
  macro sociocultural, 149
  micro sociocultural, 149
  open, definition of, 148

Vaillot, Sister Madeleine Clemence, 30

Value orientations, conflicts in health, 101
   non-Western health, 46
   Spanish-American, 124-126
   See also Case studies
Von Mering, Otto, 39, 149

White, Leslie A., 49
Wooden, Howard E., 162